THE WHITE CHAPEL

THE WHITE CHAPEL

*The "Cloistered" Life of the Disabled,
Sick & Dying Who Chose to Live in Love
Not Bitterness*

BROTHER "BERNARD FRANCIS", BS, RN,
MA, SFO

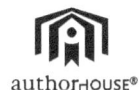

authorHOUSE®

AuthorHouse™
1663 Liberty Drive
Bloomington, IN 47403
www.authorhouse.com
Phone: 1-800-839-8640

First published by AuthorHouse   08/09/2011

ISBN: 978-1-4634-0893-0 (sc)
ISBN: 978-1-4634-0892-3 (ebk)

Library of Congress Control Number: 2011908563

Printed in the United States of America

Any people depicted in stock imagery provided by Thinkstock are models, and such images are being used for illustrative purposes only.
Certain stock imagery © Thinkstock.

This book is printed on acid-free paper.

Contents

Part I. The Art and Call of Suffering

Part II. The Science & Faith of Suffering and Death

Science

Faith

Book Reviews of: *"The White Chapel. The "Cloistered" Life of the Disabled, Sick & Dying Who Chose to Live in Love Not Bitterness. To Suffer and Pray for Him."*

"You have no idea, or maybe you do, of how timely this is. I have been struggling, just as I know you have, with trying to find what my purpose is, amidst the suffering. I know in my heart that if I just "let go" and let God direct my footsteps, in His time, that that is all I really need to do. To be reminded of doing things, the smallest things, with great love is what really matters. And that we are human beings, not human doings.

I am grateful for a kindred spirit who understands. You are a blessing.

Woman from Dayton, OH

****

"I can't tell you what a difference this made in my life! I was very discouraged having been told I would never be able to get a job due to my disabilities. You showed me I can offer up my sufferings for the salvation of others. Now I have a purpose. It drew me much closer to Christ and His love."

Man from Oregon, OH

****

"The scripture verses you gave us were a tremendous source of comfort as we read them together aloud, not just to our brother, father, husband, who was dying at that moment, but to us. Thank you!"

Family of man dying of cancer at Hospice.

****

"Brother Bernard Francis has taken the meat from quite a few references on the subject of dying, death, suffering, attaining heaven, having joy and peace even though suffering, and having a closer relationship with Christ. He has compressed these into a delightfully rich book. Some of these concepts go beyond our normal everyday thinking like "joy in suffering". But, Brother Bernard Francis helps us appreciate and understand the Saints' reasoning. He ends with Biblical verses to support it and to provide solace to the dying and their families."

Critical Care Nurse for over 30 years.

****

Comments from course attendees 1980-2008:

"I just came back from the funeral of a loved one. You gave me hope, you care, you understand."

Young USAF Sgt. After an End of life Conference in Dayton Ohio 2007.

****

"You took away our fear."

Care Giver and relative of terminal patient regarding a program at St. Richard's Catholic church.

****

"You helped us see we all need to support one another, no one is immune from the pain of losing someone you care about."

USAF doctors, nurses, medical technicians at JCAHO End of Life Program 2006-2008

****

"Death is a beautiful, sacred thing to be part of. We just need to help others through the experience."

USAF physician at conclusion of JCAHO End of life Conference 2008.

Dedication

This book is dedicated to my God: Papa, Savior, and Beloved Teacher, in gratitude and love for everything. Papa, thank you for never giving up on me, Jesus for loving me so very much and showing it so very often, and beloved Teacher, Holy Spirit, for your patience and being the best of all teachers. I also thank St. Francis for his example.

Further, it is dedicated to the two dearest sisters anyone could ever imagine, could ever hope for, pray for. They are both from France, one from Lourdes, one from Lisieux. Both died very painful physical deaths from tuberculosis, suffering nine to thirteen years from this; not to mention other sufferings, Saints Bernadette & Therese.

O how many times have I been so very close to despair, when your words entered me and I had hope and joy and love anew. May God bless you forever, and may I be able to embrace you in His House and tell you face to face how much you mean to me.

NOTE: Part I. provides much comfort from the suffering from many Saints and a review of the benefits of suffering and a discussion of how this affects ourselves and others.

Part II. Provides information on those actually going through the process of passing from this life to the next and is for caregivers primarily; with words, poems and scriptures at the end that may prove of comfort to both patient and caregiver.

I have included in the Recommended Reading and References section, those books I have read over the last 30 years that have been of help.

At the end of the book I have included reflections from on-going readings I have discovered regarding suffering and death and heaven I hope will provide additional comfort to both the person experiencing suffering and those who love them.

Foreword

Catholics are used to thinking of religious, monks, and nuns, being cloistered, living apart from society behind the walls of their monastery. In fact we are sort of subdivided into two groups: Religious and Secular. Religious live apart from society, Seculars live in society. Diocesan priests, and third order members are Seculars, and regular lay people comprise Seculars (Franciscans, Carmelites, Dominicans, Benedictines all have third orders, secular members).

Theologians see two great apostolates: an apostolate in my mind being a focus, a way to live out your spiritual life. Usually these are Service or Prayer. I believe personally that all religious orders do both, they simply stress one aspect more. Dominicans stress service and teaching, yet they still pray the Liturgy of the word and live in community when not at work serving. Carmelite and Poor Clare (Franciscan second order) Nuns pray and offer up all suffering for the salvation of the world, and although they remain within the cloister yet they serve one another by cooking, gardening, cleaning, mending, doing laundry, greeting callers, "minding the door", the porter or portress. Our master, Christ had both apostolates as well, praying & serving.

Suffering? It has long been believed by the Catholic Church that when we suffer, short term or long term, via pain or trials, we can offer this up for the benefit of souls, to be added to Christ's suffering, and aid in their redemption and salvation. It gives suffering meaning, makes it a very valuable gift. Wasn't Christ's suffering and death enough? YES! But, . . . well when you get to chapter 2. I will explain this more. And it is based largely on scripture and especially Saint Paul.

Franciscan Friars, like the rest, pray the Liturgy of the Hours (LOTH), but then they contemplate the gospels, and receive Christ into them and then take Him out to the world as they serve through nursing, social work, farming, teaching etc. After being outside serving, they return to put the concerns and needs of those they have meant, and those in the world into Christ's hands and pray for grace to grow more like Him. I have seen this as a middle of the road apostolate or a combining of both nearly equally. Yet Francis stressed the importance of prayer and contemplation first, then serving. Many Carmelites do as well. A wonderful Carmelite Discalced priest once wrote that service is like planting crops and obviously important to feed God's people. But without prayer, which is like the sun and rain, the crops will bear little fruit. Both are important and needed, but nothing is accomplished without prayer and suffering. And, as our lives are really to know and love God, then prayer and suffering seem more important.

As a professed secular Franciscan and Adjunct member of a Carmelite Secular Community I believe most of us ask ourselves where do we, as seculars, fit in? We too do both apostolates, our occasional concerns may be, am I spending too much time on prayer or on serving? We strive to pray the liturgy of the hours, contemplate and then go and serve, bring Christ to whatever work we do, whoever we serve. However, as seculars may be married (unless priests) we also have a responsibility to our spouses and children, like priests do to their parishes. We are to care for all their needs and that takes a lot of service, work, focusing on that aspect. So I myself started out doing all but my focus was service, to family and those I served at work. I would imagine members of most secular orders do much the same. We pray and serve, but our "family" asks a lot of us, requires a lot of our time, service.

The first 40 years of my life, and the first 15 as a professed secular Franciscan, my focus was service as a husband, father and a nurse practitioner. But early on I had begun the Liturgy of the Hours, initially twice a day, then three times a day, then seven times a day, as priests and religious do. You may well ask HOW? How can you be a husband, and father, and work 60 hours a week and pray seven times a day. God is wise and will help you. My family got up at 7 AM. So I got up at 4 AM. I did the Invitatory and Divine Office after showering, and after breakfast did Morning prayer—"Lauds", then hit Mass enroute to work at 630 AM. From 7-9 AM I worked, then took a 15 minute mid-morning break. My break was Mid-morning prayer, "Terce". Then I worked till 12 Noon when I did my Mid-day prayer, "Sext", just before eating. I worked till 3 PM and took a 15 minute break, for Mid-Afternoon prayer, "None". Once I was done with work I went home and changed clothes and did Evening prayer, "Vespers". Then at bedtime night-time prayer, "Compline". Each prayer took 5-10 minutes. And guess what, I never felt rushed, and I was a better husband, father, worker because of it. See I wasn't striving to be the best I could be all alone, I had God to help me.

Then in 2008 I became totally disabled. My family were grown and married and out on their own, or working full time. I was alone from 6 AM until 8 PM. Now my focus changed, it had begun to in 1999 when God told me He would be taking away nursing and giving me some of His work to do. Now my apostolate was to suffer and pray. Now I too was cloistered, I lived within the walls of my community, I was unable to drive and many days unable to walk. These days, like Bernadette, my sick bed, became my cloister, my "white chapel".

I soon learned that I was accomplishing much more by suffering and praying, then by all the successful work I had done previously. Guess what? I also found both my family and others were benefiting much more.

I have two points. My first point is that, yes, one can live a life of prayer and of service in any state of life. God will guide. My second point is that disability, illness, even when terminal, does not have to be seen as a negative, as an inability to work, to be of value. In fact, it can be, if one chooses, to be a very fulfilling life of suffering and prayer and serving all those around you and the world in a much more powerful way. You do not have to be grumpy, bitter, or suicidal; you can be excited, fulfilled, in love.

Am I alone in thinking this way? Oh no! Let's look at some Saints and their views.

"It is so beneficial, so good and so sweet to suffer."

"To obey is to love! To suffer in silence for Christ is joy!
To love sincerely is to give everything, even grief!"

When the pain became too intense, she offered it to God crying,
"Oh, my God! I offer them to you! Oh, my God! I love you!"

For four or five years of the thirteen she passed in the convent, she herself was a patient in the Infirmary: no great asset for the work of the community.

It is related that a Superioress chanced to remark on this, and said to the sickly young woman: "What are you doing there in bed, you lazy little thing?" "Why, my dear Mother, I'm doing my job." "And what's your job?" "Being ill".

For the last two years of her life she suffered terribly. "I must be a victim", she often said. Was there some connection between her vocation to suffer and the "three secrets" of Massabielle that she would never reveal to a soul? Abbe Febvre, the convent chaplain, thought there was. "He had a clear conviction", wrote his nephew Abbe Pico, "that Sister M. Bernard had a mission to live at the Mother House the lessons she received in Lourdes from the lips of Mary Immaculate: to pray, do penance, to mortify herself and to suffer for sinners." (Trochu, p. 352)

In September 1877, I said to the Sisters, "I will not last long now," and soon I became a patient in the infirmary I had helped to manage. <u>My bed became "my little white chapel." Then it became my cross. Eventually it became a crucifix, when I could only lie on it and suffer. (The cover is a rendition of a similar bed with holy cards pinned on the sheets to meditate and pray, and a Breviary lying on the bed.)</u>

"Pass on Creature, God alone is sufficient. Christ is mine still."

"Suffering is my job."

"Let us work only for God."

"My God take my heart and make it burn (with love for You)."

"It's for the good Lord. We have to suffer for Him; He suffered enough for us."

"Tell Your Guardian angel to bring your messages to Jesus in the tabernacle."

Rene Laurentin, translated by John Lynch, SM and Ronald DesRosiers, SM. <u>Bernadette in Her Own Words.</u> Pauline Books and Media, Boston; 2000.

"O Jesus and Mary, let my entire consolation in this world be to love you and to suffer for sinners."

"I must die to myself continually and accept trials without complaining. I work, I suffer and I love with no other witnesses than His heart. Anyone who is not prepared to suffer all for the Beloved and to do His will in all things is not worthy of the sweet name of Friend, for here below, love without suffering does not exist."

"I shall spend every moment loving. One who loves does not notice her trials; or perhaps more accurately, she is able to love them."

O my Mother, to you I sacrifice all other attachments so that my heart may belong entirely to you and my Jesus."

"I shall do everything for heaven, my true home. There I shall find my mother in all the splendor of her glory. I shall delight with her in the joy of Jesus Himself in perfect safety."

"From this moment on, anything concerning me is no longer of any interest to me. I must belong entirely to God and God alone. Never to myself."

"Love overcomes, love delights."

"Jesus my God, I love You above all things."

"Let the crucifix be not only in my eyes and on my breast, but in my heart. O Jesus! Release all my affections and draw them upwards. Let my crucified heart sink forever into Yours and bury itself in the mysterious wound made by the entry of the lance."

"O my God, I beg You, by Your loneliness, not that You may spare me affliction, but that You may not abandon me in it. When I encounter affliction, teach me to see You in it as my sole Comforter. Let affliction strengthen my faith, fortify my hope, and purify my love. Grant me the grace to see Your hand in my affliction, and to desire no other comforter but you."

"Jesus keep me under the standard of Your Cross. May the crucifix not be just something I wear, something I look at, but let it be alive in my heart. Let me be transformed into a living crucifixion, in union with You in the Eucharist. By meditating on Your life and the most intimate feelings of Your heart, let me draw souls to You from on high on this cross where Your love holds me forever."

From: The Private Notes of Saint Bernadette of Lourdes p29. A Holy Life—Patricia A McEachern

All of above quotes from: St. Bernadette

"It is in suffering and not in rejoicing that true love is proven; a day without the Cross is lost for heaven. Don't cease to suffer for a moment and you will not cease to love. Joy is to be found only in suffering and in suffering without any consolation! Your aridities (dryness), your sufferings, these are something to offer Jesus both for Himself and for souls. Love is repaid only by love." "What a joy to be humbled; it is the only thing that makes saints." St. Therese Letter to Celine

"Let us love Him enough to suffer for Him all that He wills, even spiritual pains, aridities, anxieties, apparent coldness . . . Ah,

here is great love, to love Jesus without feeling the sweetness
of His love . . . this is martyrdom . . . Well then let us die as
martyrs!"
"Is there a greater joy than to suffer for Your love, O my God?
The more intense and the more hidden the suffering the more
you value it."
St. Therese's Story of a Soul

"Speak, my Jesus! Speak . . . what must I do to console
You?" And Jesus answers: "What I want from you, faithful
Soul, is LOVE . . . Humble love that reduces self to
nothing . . . generous love that forgets self."

"We share the chalice of Jesus' Sufferings; but how sweet it will
be for us one day to hear . . . "You are those who have stood
by me in my trials, and I confer on you, just as my father has
conferred on me, a Kingdom." Letter to Sr. Genevieve

"During the short moments that remain to us, let us not lose our
time . . . let us save souls . . . souls are being lost like flakes
of snow, and Jesus weeps, and we . . . we are thinking of our
sorrow without consoling our beloved . . . Oh let us live for
souls."

"There is only Jesus. Let us love Him, then, unto folly: let us
save souls for Him. Jesus is asking us to quench His thirst by
giving Him souls, the souls of priests especially. Our mission is
to forget ourselves and to reduce ourselves to nothing . . . We
are so insignificant . . . and yet Jesus wills that the salvation of
souls depends on the sacrifices of our love. He is begging souls
from us . . . Ah, let us understand His look!"

"Take flight to the All of your heart with the wings of humility,
simplicity and love."

"The God of strength loves to show His power by making use of
nothing."

From: Sermon in a Sentence, John P. McClernon

"I feel we must tread the same road, the road of suffering and love. When I myself have reached the port, I will teach you how best to sail the world's tempestuous sea—with the self-abandonment of a child well aware of its father's love, and of His vigilance in the hour of danger."

"I Turn to God and to all of His Saints and I thank them notwithstanding (for the feelings of being discouraged and forsaken); I believe they want to see how far I will trust them. But the words of Job have not entered my heart in vain: "Even if God should kill me, I would still trust Him." (Job 13:15). I admit that it has taken a long time to arrive at this degree of self-abandonment; but I have reached it now, and it is our Lord Himself who has brought me there."

"I desire neither death nor life. Were our Lord to offer me my choice, I would not choose. I only will what He wills, and I am pleased with whatever He does. I have no fear of the last struggle, or of any pain, however great, which my illness may bring. God has always been my help; He has led me by the hand since I was a child and I count on Him now. Even though suffering should reach its furthest limits I am certain He will never forsake me."
Therese of Lisieux—In My Own Words, by Judith Bauer, Ligori Press

"Let us love Him enough to suffer for Him all that He wills, even spiritual pains, aridities, anxieties, apparent coldness . . . Ah, here is great love, to love Jesus without feeling the sweetness of His love . . . this is martyrdom . . . Well then let us die as martyrs!" Letter to Celine

"Is there a greater joy than to suffer for Your love, O my God? The more intense and the more hidden the suffering the more you value it." Story of a Soul

"We share the chalice of Jesus' Sufferings; but how sweet it will be for us one day to hear . . . 'You are those who have stood by me in my trials, and I confer on you, just as my father has conferred on me, a Kingdom.'" Letter to Sr. Genevieve

"The God of strength loves to show His power by making use of nothing."
Sermon in a Sentence, John P. McClernon

"I desire neither death nor life. Were our Lord to offer me my choice, I would not choose. I only will what He wills, and I am pleased with whatever He does. I have no fear of the last struggle, or of any pain, however great, which my illness may bring. God has always been my help; He has led me by the hand since I was a child and I count on Him now. Even though suffering should reach its furthest limits I am certain He will never forsake me."
Therese of Lisieux—In My Own Words, by Judith Bauer, Ligori Press

A Sister was speaking to her about the happiness of heaven: Therese interrupted saying: "It is not that which attracts me." The Sister asked, "what is it then?" Therese replied: "O! it is Love! To love, to be beloved, and to come back to earth to make Love loved."
Tan-Thoughts of St. Therese

"Jesus, Jesus! If it be so sweet to desire Thy love, what will it be to possess and enjoy it forever!"
Tan-Thoughts of St. Therese

All The above quotes by St. Therese of Lisieux

"Pray, and then pray more."

"Surround yourself with the Saints. Seek the Holy Soul's prayers."

<u>"Speak words of love to the Beloved."</u>

<u>"With joy I have chosen the way of suffering! I shall enjoy all persecutions in the name of the Savior for as long as it shall please Him to send them."</u>

<u>See Christ on the Cross, "You see how much I suffered for you? Do not be sad then that you must suffer for me."</u>

All of above quotes from: St. Catherine of Siena

Blessed Raymond of Capua, translated by George Lamb. <u>The Life of St. Catherine of Siena</u>. Tan Books and Publishers, Rockford; 2003.

"I bear on my body the marks of Jesus." Gal 6:17

"Now I rejoice in my sufferings for your sake, and in my flesh I complete what is lacking in Christ's afflictions for the sake of His body, that is, the church." Col 1:24

"Even if I am poured as a libation upon the sacrificial offering of your faith, I am glad and rejoice with you all." Phil 2:17

"I appeal to you therefore, brethren, by the mercies of God, to present your bodies as a living sacrifice, holy & acceptable to God, which is your spiritual worship." Rom 12:1

"Brothers, I beg you through the mercy of God to <u>offer your bodies as a living sacrifice holy and acceptable to God,</u> your spiritual worship. Do not conform yourselves to this age but <u>be transformed by the renewal of your mind, so that you may judge what is God's will</u>, what is good, pleasing and perfect." Romans 12:1-2

"Companions with Him in His suffering, you will share in his overflowing happiness." Cor. 1:7

"Strict justice requires that God will provide relief to you who are sorely tried, as well as to us, when the Lord Jesus is revealed from heaven with His mighty angels, on the day when He comes, to be glorified in His holy ones and adored by all who believe. 2 Thessalonians. 1:6-10

All of above quotes from: St. Paul

Why are you cast down, my soul, why groan within me?
Hope in God: I will praise Him still, my Savior and my God.
Ps 42

You do not ask for sacrifice and offerings, but an open ear,
You do not ask for holocausts and victim. Instead, here am I.
Ps 40

I rejoiced when I heard the say: Let us go to God's house!
And now our feet are standing within your gates O Jerusalem!
Ps 122

Companions with Him in suffering, you will share His
overflowing happiness. 2 Corinthians 1:7

Regarding this book:

"I am nothing. A pencil can do nothing by itself. It needs a hand, strength and a mind to use it. God so often chooses the least worthy (St. Francis' words), the most ignorant (St. Bernadette's words). Then His power and His will use this instrument to accomplish His purpose out of love for His children. Then His love is seen and embraced. It is all God. How blessed to be an instrument in His hand. How blessed to know and love Him and to be content whether in His hand, or lying on the table awaiting His will." Bro. Bernard Francis, SFO

Introduction

Can suffering have a purpose?

I am a Catholic, born and raised in the Church from my birth in 1950, yet I was not baptized until 1971. My father said to, "Go to all the Churches and become a member of the one that . . . well you'll know. The one that is right for you."

In 1970 I began searching for God. I wanted to really know Him. I prayed, attended a retreat and found Him in a Paul-like way. Some of us need a lightning bolt to the head to get our attention. I became a Catholic in 1971.

In 1987 I began the journey to becoming a Secular Franciscan and with Francis leading, found out about mysticism in a hands-on way from him. I professed in 1990.

In 1999 I had grown in my relationship with God and asked Him, "What is it you want me to do." I was used to talking with Him throughout my day and although it took 8 weeks for me to first learn to listen and to hear Him in 1971, by now He usually answered in minutes. His answer, "I want you to quit the United States Air Force, now. And in a while I will have you stop nursing."

I had been a nurse 19 years and an Air Force Nurse ten. I loved both. But nursing, it gave me a sense of worth I had never felt as a child or young man. In nursing I forgot about me while thinking just about others. I didn't like me, because most of my life as a child no one had. My parents were impaired by alcohol, my brother 10 years older.

I was afraid and I asked Him, "Why would You take away nursing from my life?"

And He replied, "Because you don't need it anymore. I led you to do it for all these years to like yourself a bit and to find that I love you. Now I can use you to do my work."

I kept working, daily, fearfully asking, "Do you want me to quit today?" And almost with a subdued chuckle I would hear, "No, not today." Or nothing.

Then in 2006 a disease of the inner ear I had since 1995, undiagnosed until 2003, began to worsen despite every effort imaginable and soon after I developed it in both ears which ruled out most viable options surgically.

By 2008 I was unable to walk without a walker and could not safely drive any vehicle. I became disabled, and unable to provide financially for my family in any way for about a year when disability benefits finally began.

In 2005 I received a rather shocking addition to my life as a mystic. By the way all Catholics are mystics.

St. Bonaventure, St. John of the Cross and St. Teresa of Avila,
all doctors of the Catholic Church on Mysticism,
believed that all are called to be mystics.
That is, all are called to a mystical, intimate relationship,
with Christ.

Catechism 2014—"Spiritual progress tends toward ever more intimate union with Christ.

This union is called "mystical" because it participates in the mystery of Christ through the sacraments—"the holy mysteries"—and, in Him, in the mystery of the Holy Trinity.

God calls us all to intimate union with Him, even if the special graces or extraordinary signs of this mystical life are granted only to some for the sake of manifesting the gratuitous gift given to all."

My experience was so shocking I went for help thinking I might be going crazy. I found excellent spiritual directors who helped me and directed my reading.

In 2006, it was if St. Francis and Jesus put me into a little French Nun's (Therese of Lisieux) hands and said, "She will walk with you to heaven." Our Lord, knows I am thick headed, and still carry emotional wounds, and need a lot of help and supervision. As I look back I find it another example of God's love for us.

As Therese said, "His love for us is more tender than that of a mother for her child."

When I was a child of about five, at one point I was told I might be without a family the next morning, and if that happened, I should walk from Toledo, Ohio to Omaha, Nebraska and a priest, Father Flanagan, would take care of me. I was so scared!

That night I saw what appeared to be a very small nun in a very big habit in the corner of my room praying, this scared me at first but then I thought, "Well Nuns are good and if she is praying for me, I guess I'll be all right." From that time on my family life slowly improved. My parents quit drinking in 1963 & became mirrors of Christ.

For almost 40 years I would ask and think who that nun was, and now I am sure that little nun was Bernadette. So now two French sisters, how good our God is.

In 2008-09 the disease reached a point where 4 out of 7 days I was bedridden and really never felt good. I had severe ringing in my ears constantly and was going deaf despite hearing aids. My balance essentially gone, I never knew from second to second when I would fall flat on my face or down stairs.

At the same time I was going through emotional, mental and spiritual hurts. I even had two family members accuse me of, "faking it all and being a lazy, fat bum."

God used Therese and Bernadette and others, He directed me to read, to see suffering, of any kind, can have a purpose, and can even become, (and in 1999 I would have found this impossible to believe), "sweet and something to be greatly desired." Not in a masochistic way but in a beautiful way associated with falling in love more and more deeply with Christ. Knowing Him through suffering as He had suffered.

Today as I sat at my table I thought. I have come to the point of desiring suffering and martyrdom and loving Him more than I ever would have believed possible. And what would have caused me to consider suicide in 1970, now is a reason to rejoice.

I know I am not alone, being in nursing 40 years clued me into that. So I decided to write this book to perhaps give a bit of that same hope and joy to others and to refer them to at least a few experts on this.

I need to say one more thing. My youngest daughter at 13 developed leukemia. She fought, and won, a long hard five year battle. During chemotherapy when she was ill once she turned in bed and said to me, "You know what makes all this worthwhile?" I replied, "No." She said, "Because everything they try on me, its results, help them treat all the patients after me better. Because I am suffering all who follow will suffer less and do better."

Thoughts from St. Therese of Lisieux from a presentation on Victim Souls I did in 2006

- Victim soul: One who lives with one thought in mind; that of consoling God by redeeming souls. Souls are redeemed by sacrifice. The sacrifice of one's self, of never belonging to oneself again, a life of constant giving. Becoming all things to all people.
- To be a victim of divine justice, by suffering for souls' redemption, but even more to suffer for others to bring them to Christ, and to be a victim of merciful love. To be a victim of merciful love is to turn from happiness in this world, dying to all in this world. To suffer for others out of love of them and Christ, to take on Jesus' crown of thorns and cross and give Him rest and encouragement. He is consoled by love; and by enkindling love in hearts where it was extinguished.
- To love Christ. He loves so many but His love is rejected. Can we not accept His love, to be empty vessels for Him, allowing Him to pour His pent up love into us.
- To be consumed in the fire of God's love by abandonment and surrender to Him. To at last die for His love fills us, consumes us, and makes us one with Him.
- A life of becoming the heart, the love of the church.
- To work for His love alone with the one purpose of pleasing Him, consoling His Sacred heart, and saving souls who will love Him eternally.
- First aim at ever increasing humility, to clear one's heart of all encumbrances, to keep it empty of confidence in self and all vain seeking after creatures. To be always afar off, in lowliness, in nothingness. To more and more sincerely

acknowledge our littleness, our nothingness. Second, more and more <u>abandon oneself like the little child who sleeps without fear in His Father's arms.</u> Abandonment alone surrenders the soul into the arms of Jesus, allowing His love to act freely to the full extent of its force.

Prayer becomes more listening than talking.

- Depend solely on His love. Knowing we can do nothing. Hoping, trusting, His merciful love will provide all the virtue we need. I desire to be a Saint but am helpless, God be my Sanctity.
- The victim soul draws life from Holy Communion. Daily communion is the bread that gives us strength to do His will, to become one with Him.
- I do not fear suffering, for as it increases God will increase my patience.

There are so many books I have read on Therese I could not find all the references—see Recommended Reading.

- **St. Gertrude** "God speaks to whom He pleases, and makes no distinction . . . unless indeed it be to give more abundantly to the weaker when they deserve it by humility and devotion." From the life of St. Gertrude the Great, by TAN
- **St. Margaret Mary** "I come to offer myself to You in the quality of victim . . . to immolate me on the altar of Your amiable heart." From Devotion to the Sacred Heart, TAN
- **St. Francis of Assisi**—The first of the stigmatists, one who bears the wounds of Christ's Passion and Crucifixion. He loved Christ and wanted to share in His passion. From the Omnibus of Sources on St. Francis.
- **St. Pio** "For some time past I have felt the need to offer myself to the Lord as a victim for poor sinners and for the souls in purgatory. This desire has been growing continually in my heart." From Padre Pio, The True Story.
- **Sr. Josefa Menendez** "When victim-souls contemplate Him, He unveils the immensity of His love for souls and

the grief with which the loss of sinners fills Him. The sight of this breaks their hearts, and their longing to console Christ is not satisfied with mere words of love; it stirs up their zeal. At whatever price, they will win souls to Him, and He kindles this zeal still more. It is the love of the Sacred Heart itself, communicating to them, with which they love sinners; love which gives them a superhuman endurance." From The Way of Divine Love, by TAN

- **St. Faustina** "By saying the Chaplet (of Divine Mercy) you are bringing humankind closer to me. I often felt the passion of Our Lord present in my body, although this was imperceptible to others, and I rejoiced in it because Jesus wanted it so. These sufferings set my soul afire with love for God and for immortal souls. Love endures everything, love is stronger than death, love fears nothing." From the Diary of St. Faustina

- **St. Bernadette** "Why should I be prideful. He chose me after all because I was the most stupid person He could find." (So His workings would be obvious.)

I am a great believer in this. So many saints, especially my dear Francis, thought they had been chosen because they were the least likely to ever do any good. So people seeing their actions would say, "God must be working in that person because there is no other way they could do that. That is from God."

In reading extensively I have found two types of victim souls: I. The person who offers themselves to suffer God's judgment in behalf of others.

II. The person who offers themselves up as a victim to God's love, to accept His pent up love, as so very few on this earth accept God's love for them either out of a feeling of guilt or unworthiness, or indifference. I see little difference, both suffer out of love.

All of us can offer up our sufferings, to be united with Christ's, for the salvation and redemption of the poor souls and sinners everywhere. Some may become like Saints, victim souls.

"To offer oneself as a victim to Divine Love is not to offer oneself to sweetness, to consolation; but to every anguish, every bitterness, for love lives only by sacrifice; and the more a soul wills to be surrendered to Love, the more must she be surrendered to suffering." Therese of Lisieux Story of a Soul, Thoughts of Saint Therese by TAN.

There are many books that deal with victim souls. One of my favorites is the book by

Michael Freze SFO, "They Bore The Wounds of Christ." Also, "The Way of Divine Love." By Sister Josepha Menendez & the books on Padre Pio, Bernadette & Therese.

I personally have often thought the first victim soul after Jesus was Our Lady.

I am not a theologian. I am a very little soul whom God is leading on a journey. I believe He gives us tasks to do and that I am to talk to others about: 1) Interceding for the world, 2) devotion for the poor souls in purgatory and 3) growing into a more intimate union with God, becoming mystics. 4) And that Our Lady would have me urge all to grow in: Poverty, Prayer and Penance. How does one grow in poverty, by never allowing "things" to possess you, only allowing God to possess you.

By the way powerful weapons to use in interceding for others is to offer up your pain, and should God ask, to agree to become a victim soul, one who suffers for them.

Chapter 1

Are You Being Called to Suffer?
Can anyone offer up suffering?

So are you being called to suffer? I found the book by Michael Freze, "They Bore the Wounds of Christ." It was very beneficial in understanding mysticism and the concept of victim souls. My spiritual director suggested I read the works of St. Teresa of Avila, a Carmelite who reformed her order. She was helped by St. John of the Cross and there is an excellent book, "Fire Within." By Father Thomas Dubay, it combines their teachings and is good as well for those new to all this. Also St. Bonaventure, a Franciscan, actually wrote on this and his works were used by St. John of the Cross in his teaching.

First, if you have an experience, or feelings, that God wants you to grow in His relationship with you, seek a good spiritual director. Not all priests are gifted in this way. My experience is that all my best spiritual directors were prior monks now diocesan priests. Most will know if they are gifted in being able to guide souls in mysticism.

Notice the first thing I did was go on retreat and talk to God and try and discern His will and call ahead and arrange a meeting with two very mature Catholics and secular Franciscans who had experience in this area and a Bishop who worked with them.

They and I prayed I would find excellent spiritual directors and I did through asking around my parish.

I received excellent advice and one bit was to not discuss this with anyone except my spiritual director and close family members who already knew, i.e. my wife. My best director told me after a two hour talk, "This is what I feel God is calling you to do . . . and that means you have gone from a harmless, mediocre Catholic, to one on fire for God.

You are now a threat to the other side and when the evil one finds out, well it will be challenging."

It was funny but I had come in contact with and knew of another excellent spiritual director. I had by pure accident requested an appointment with him and it wound up it was 3 hours later. He confirmed everything the first director told me. This was a great reassurance.

I believe it was Teresa of Avila who said many things that helped me greatly: 1) a poor spiritual director can cause much harm. 2) God is a gentleman. He always asks if you would be a victim soul, or suffer, for Him.

I believe she also said that true calling initially fills one with fear then peace, the opposite is true when the enemy is involved, there is initial peace then unrest.

I would echo the advice of my director, read her works. She is the #1 doctor on mysticism.

By the way another way to track down a good director is to locate the minister of a secular order, there are Franciscan, Carmelite, Dominican and Benedictine third—lay orders. They often have had to learn who good spiritual directors are so are good resources, as are priests and Nuns.

So, if you have a feeling you are being asked to follow this journey, find a good spiritual director, and read St. Teresa.

But am I worthy? See below.

Can anyone offer up their sufferings?

Yes, the Catholic Church has long taught if you suffer, offer it up for the poor souls in purgatory, the conversion of sinners, the sanctification and purification of priests.

What does this do? In my experience you will see its effects, you will grow in virtue and as time goes by you will be sought out for prayer. As one director said, God will direct people to you, you don't have to worry about it.

But I am not worthy? This was a major problem for me. I truly knew if I were God and formed a line of potential saints, I would be the last one in the line, maybe taking lunch orders. Read the lives of the Saints. Be open, pray and ask God's help.

Your Father does not want you to go astray. Of course one has to listen. This means instead of going to church and unloading all of our past sins and needs for hours, we say, "Your servant is listening." And we shut up, for as long as it takes. The first time (in 1971) it took me eight weeks, 45 minutes a day. In 2005, He contacted me.

It seems to me all of the saints felt unworthy. Remember Bernadette's quote, *"Mary picked me because I was the most ignorant person she could find."* Francis said something very similar: *"I am in this generation the most wretched creature; the most utterly useless and destitute. You have chosen the most foolish to put the wise to shame, the weakest to put the strong to shame. You have chosen what in this world is lowborn & insignificant and treated with contempt, the littlest nothing, . . ."*

None of us are worthy. That is not the point. What Therese said, **IS** the point, "He chooses who He will."

Teresa of Avila, her spiritual mother, so to speak, said, all are called to contemplation but our progress is solely in the hands of God. Our job is to sincerely surrender to Him and wait, even if it takes a lifetime.

Some of us in this life will simply offer up our sufferings that occur, throughout the course of life, for others and in doing this gain graces and forgiveness for others. But, there are a few who will be asked by God to suffer, like Christ, for the salvation and redemption of His children.

Are you one He is calling to do this in a regular way, or a bigger way like some. I believe Therese and Bernadette and Padre Pio were victim souls as was St. Francis and St. Catherine of Siena. You will have to listen and when you hear His calm, quiet voice within you, answer out of love. Anything that accomplishes anything is always done out of love.

"Just as a torrent sweeps along with it unto the depths of the sea whatsoever it encounters on its course, even so, my Jesus, does the soul which plunges into the boundless ocean of Thy love draw after her all her treasures. Lord, Thou knowest that for Thee these treasures are the souls it has pleased Thee to unite to mine."

Therese of Lisieux Story of a Soul, Thoughts of Saint Therese TAN Books.

Chapter 2

What are the Types of Suffering— Which are Easiest?

I have never really seen this delineated, spelled out. But I believe there are four kinds of suffering: 1) Physical 2) Mental 3) Emotional 4) Spiritual. Which is hardest, I suspect this is individual. God has made each of us unique. For me I found they were in that order; physical was easiest, though I did not think so at first. Spiritual seems THE hardest. Be of good cheer. God will slowly, with perfect timing guide you, and He will prepare you so you are ready for the next level when He knows it is the best time. You may not feel ready but He knows you infinitely better than you know yourself.

Again, I personally felt Thomas Dubay's book, "Fire Within." And the writings of Saint Teresa of Avila and St. John of the Cross. Tremendous helps. Really, like the only dim light in a stormy black night that really scared you. It was as if they took my hand and guided me and all was okay. And I found it interesting that until I needed to understand John of the Cross, I could not. God had to get me to that point.

So are you passing a kidney stone? Are you having a gallbladder attack? Do you have arthritis? Do you have cancer, or Crohn's disease, a steroid injection into a severely painful joint, dental work, stubbed toe—whatever physical pain be it: short, long-lived, one-time or repeating, you can pray, "Father, I offer up my suffering for the poor souls, the conversion of sinners and the sanctification of priests.", as He leads.

May I share something very intimate with you? Do you realize that when you suffer pain you become ONE with Jesus on the Cross. You will soon find that there is no more intimate relationship in the world. I cannot feel my wife's headache. She cannot feel my severe nausea. Yet we can share in what Christ

Himself suffered for us. As if we were occupying the same body at the same time. God can use this suffering, as He did Jesus', for the salvation of the world. I have gotten in arguments with friends over this. Wasn't Jesus sacrifice enough? The answer I believe is <u>yes</u>. Well then why do we have to suffer and how can it be redemptive? Because God, our Father, Creator, the Boss chooses it to be. Why? If I were God and being honest, I probably would not want to create a bunch of robots that rushed to fulfill my every wish. I would rather have children who loved me, who wanted to be like me. So, I would have to give them free will. Then they could choose to love me. (Oh by-the-way you can say no to offering up suffering, to this intimacy with God.) I would also want them to share in my work.

When I was a little boy I went into my father's workshop. He was a wood craftsman after retirement and had many projects for customers. He could see I dearly wanted to help Him, because I loved him. And so, because he loved me he said, "Would you help me? I really need someone to take all these blocks of wood and sand them for me so the corners are smooth. Here let me show you how." So he gave me some sandpaper and a box to put them in. I was in heaven, I worked so hard all day. He said as he was getting ready to lock up. "That is the best job of sanding I have ever seen, thank you. I'll have some more in a few days, will you help me?" I told him, "Sure Dad." And we went in to supper. Years later I learned the blocks of wood were left over pieces that were to be thrown away. But my Father and I worked together, we would stop and glance each other's way and smile, we shared a task. I believe our heavenly Father is no different, so He gives us work we can help with; because He chooses to, because He loves us so very dearly. And because He loves us, our suffering does matter greatly to Him, and He will use it to help others and ourselves and loved ones. I have seen it over 40 years in the field of nursing as a Catholic.

<u>From Volume II, Lenten Season, of the Liturgy of the Hours, By Saint Irenaeus, Bishop:</u>

. . . Nor did the Lord need our service. He commanded us to follow Him, but His was the gift of salvation. To follow the Savior is to share in salvation; to follow the light is to enjoy the

light. Those who are in the light do not illuminate the light but are themselves illuminated and enlightened by the light. They add nothing to the light; rather, they are beneficiaries, for they are enlightened by the light.

The same is true of service to God: it adds nothing to God, nor does God need the service of man. Rather, He gives life and immortality and eternal glory to those who follow and serve Him. He confers a benefit on His servants in return for their service and on His followers in return for their loyalty, but He receives no benefit from them. He is rich, perfect and in need of nothing.

The reason why God requires service from man is this: because He is good and merciful He desires to confer benefits on those who persevere in His service. In proportion to God's need of nothing is man's need for communion with God.

This is the glory of man: to persevere and remain in the service of God. For this reason the Lord told His disciples: "You did not choose me but I chose you." He meant that His disciples did not glorify Him by following Him, but in following the Son of God they were glorified by Him. As He said, "I wish that where I am they also may be, that they might see my glory." To follow in Christ's footsteps, to offer up our suffering and prayers for God's children, to by serving and loving help them to know His love.

He loves us, with a tender, merciful, limitless love. ". . . an abyss of love that cannot be measured so big that all my love is like a tear drop in the ocean of His love." as Therese would say.

Have you thought about, or are you already in the position where due to weakness or paralysis you can't bathe yourself, have lost bowel and or bladder control and have to have nursing personnel or even your own family clean you? I recently thought about this becoming a possibility in my own life and was . . . upset. Then I thought about Jesus, stripped of His clothing and nailed to the Cross and lifted up for all the world to see. He understands. When you have this problem you share intimately in what He suffered. So why not add it to His suffering for the salvation and redemption of others.

What if you can no longer speak? What if you can no longer think? I too have experienced this due to medication side effects. It can be embarrassing as well. To perhaps recognize a loved one but no longer verbally communicate could be very frustrating and embarrassing and discouraging. But remember, "Now I rejoice in my sufferings for your sake, and in my flesh I complete what is lacking in Christ's afflictions for the sake of His body, that is, the church." Paul, Col 1:24.

I realized that Jesus may have not had Meniere's disease, TB, HIV, confusion, inability to talk. But He can use our sufferings to "complete what is lacking in Christ's afflictions" when you are willing to offer up your sufferings, these sufferings, to Him out of passionate (ardent, fervent, enthusiastic) love for Him.

What about <u>Emotional pain</u>, well one night one of my children looked at me and said, "You are a fat, useless, pathetic cripple, addicted to pain medication." (I wasn't on any?) Months before this person said, "You're faking everything. There's nothing wrong with you. You don't have Meniere's, and the ringing, pain, nausea, spinning, imbalance, deafness that comes with that."

About a month later another child told me, "You know for a long time I thought perhaps you were lying or exaggerating. Then I prayed and realized these negative thoughts were from Satan. I know you Dad. You have never been like that and I don't believe ever could be. But I wanted to tell you I'm sorry for even thinking it for a while."

<u>Mental Pain.</u> My medication at one point so affected me that I would start to pray the "Our Father", and two hours later could remember what came next. Frustrating? Yes. Fear inspiring? Could be if you dwell on, "I'm losing it, I'll be a confused nut job any day now." But you can offer this up. "Lord, I offer the pain my forgetfulness causes me."

<u>Spiritual pain</u>. John of the Cross and again Teresa of Avila have great advice. You have developed an intimate, passionate, great relationship with Christ and are living and experience things you never dreamed possible, wonderful! As Therese and Pio talked about great, "consolations" unnecessary for those who love deeply. Then what if He, as Therese says, "Hides." You can't seem to find God. You're cut off from Him. You may even feel He hates you, for all those mistakes you made. Personally I have come to believe that when you don't see Him, He is hiding right behind you, watching over you and watching to see if you

love Him enough without consolations, without any proof He exists or loves you. That is Love. As Therese and Bernadette said, "Love without suffering is impossible in this life." Padre Pio said consolations were just candy for babies, real love didn't need them.

When I dated my wife I thought I was in love. When we got married I thought I was in love. When I let her sleep and changed the baby's dirty diapers at 3 AM, and didn't tell her, I just let her sleep, all even though I was exhausted from work; then I knew I loved her. When I fell asleep and awoke kneeling in the refrigerator, baby bottle in hand, holding a child I had walked the floors with for hours who had chickenpox, that was true love. True love is dying to self, enduring suffering for the one you love.

Sometimes the enemy's attacks come, become more . . . visible, physical. That I leave you to talk to a priest about or read about in the lives of Saints like Padre Pio or Sr. Josepha Menendez.

Chapter 3

How Will Your Family Feel?
Are There Stages in Acceptance?

I can only share my experience. My daughters, who have always been able to wheedle information out of me, were impressed and thought it cool. They began to seek God more and grow in their relationship with Him. They came to me with prayer requests, because, oh God really hears prayers offered up in suffering. This became obvious to all of us who knew.

My wife became very upset and angry initially. Why you? I love you, I don't want you to suffer. It's not fair. I had to share with her the benefits to me and share my joy, until she could see God's blessings being poured out on those we loved.

Are there stages in acceptance. My family showed me some. The first was, "What?" (Is Dad nuts? What is he trying for, "martyr of the year"?) The next, after I had explained as I learned, was, "That sounds kind of neat." The third was, "So could you pray about this?" and most requests were real life threatening situations in friends etc. And it caused them to examine their own faith and prayer life.

One very mature Christian friend, passionately in love with Christ said to me, "I wish I could be a saint. I wish I could experience mystical experiences." I said, "Have you asked? Have you asked and then believed He might want to do this, to use you in this way, and so listened for His answer, no matter how long it takes or what He says? He tends to use the most worthless. Oh He used brilliant people. But many Saints were stupid, stubborn, playboys, and all were sinners. If He has used Francis of Assisi, Augustine, Bernadette, and me, He can use you."

She is now I believe experiencing mystical graces and will far more. She opened the door a crack and He got in. That's all it takes. Just saying, "What if . . . ?" And really being open to Him, WOW! Then He can use you and most likely will.

So, although this information may be of tremendous help to you the patient, and eventually to you the care giver, it may not be well accepted at first.

Chapter 4

Chores and Their Benefits

So, Most days I get sick around 10 AM. So I get up at 5 or 6 AM, do my Liturgy of the Hours: Invitatory, Morning Prayers, and Mid-morning prayers, then I go to Communion. 10 AM I go to bed for anywhere from 2-8 hours. In between if I can walk without falling, I do the dishes, do the laundry, write letters to friends and to others who are sick. Then its back to prayers and devotions until my wife gets home around 8-9 PM. She is a nurse and works 12+ hour shifts. So My day looks like this:

0500 Prayers and shower
0530 Invitatory and Breakfast
0600 Meds, Office of Readings and Morning Prayer
0630 Prayers and chores. Wife off to work.
0830 Mass, friends or my son take me, or deacon brings communion later in the day.
0930 Mid-morning Prayer, chores, personal prayers and intercessions for others.
1200 Mid-day prayer and lunch. Spiritual reading, lives of the saints.
1400 Meds
1500 Mid afternoon prayer, Rosaries, chaplets etc. chores.
1800 Evening prayer. 1700: Supper. Spiritual reading, lives of the saints.
2100 Meds. Wife gets home. The cloistered lay monk disappears and the husband reappears. At bedtime, 10 PM, I finish with Night Prayer and an examination of conscience. Some bad days, everything is done while in bed.

In a monastery the monks or nuns spend their days usually like this, prayers interspersed with helping others. We can too even if we are married, even if we have children. People always take precedence over prayer, <u>except</u> say some prayers for help and grace early, before people are awake, so you can help them better.

Does living like this, does focusing on Christ, does loving Him more than anyone else, shortchange or lessen your doing your duty as husband, wife, mother, father? I battled with this and others do as well. When I had been married for about a year, this was about 4 years after I met Christ and had a personal relationship with Him, I was shocked to discover that I now loved Him more than my wife. I remember I was working in the garage and praying/thinking. Oh my gosh, was this good or bad, should I change in some way . . . ? The answer: NO! When we take marriage vows they are as binding as the sacred vows of priests and religious. But my wife now could be loved by me, a nice guy with problems and faults, or be loved by this same guy filled with Jesus Christ.

How much difference in love would she profit by? An infinite amount! As I died more and more to me and the world, and lived more and more for Christ, He was able to love my wife and children more through me, I became a much better spouse and parent.

Both my wife and youngest daughter see this very clearly. My oldest daughter and youngest son, I think have a gut feeling I am a better father. Old friends and even strangers I meet seem to be attracted to me more regarding, well, one said, "What's different about you?" I said "What do you mean?" They said when you come into a room there is a peace and joy that is wonderful, even if you don't say anything, it just flows out of you." Often I say, "Oh! That would be Jesus Christ, not me. We're very close," then we have awesome talks.

So what about chores? Can they be used, can every day work and labor be used, offered up? Yes!

When I do the dishes, laundry, clean the bathrooms, etc., I pray, "O Lord, as I wash away these stains, please wash away the stains of sin from your children, that we may be with you in heaven one day. I offer up all I am doing for this."

What about devotions rosaries, chaplets? Oh yes, I have found you can say "focused rosaries." If you are praying for someone or a group apply each mystery of the rosary to them.

For instance, The first Joyful mystery is the Annunciation, O Lord, help _____, and all of us your children, to pray like Mary, "Be it done to me according to Your will." And mean it, and see them praying this way. Dying completely to self and wanting His will alone. WOW! This appears quite powerful.

So chores and work and actions can also be quite effective in helping others, in sharing in Christ's work. How great!

Both Teresa of Avila and Therese of Lisieux talk about throwing straw on the embers of love. They have caused me to do it just through association, . . . and praying for it. Several times a day just pause and say, "I love You God." "O Papa, I love you so very much!" "Jesus, You are everything to me, I love You!" Even, and get this, even if you don't feel like it. Grumpy, judgmental, frustrated, tired, don't feel any love is left? Do it anyway. Then, feel His love flow over you. I use beads called, "St. Therese's Good Deed Beads." I use them to remind me to tell God 20 times each day that I love Him so.

Chapter 5

Various Devotions

I cannot stress enough you must discern through prayer, spiritual directors, reading, and LISTENING what it is God wants of you, and then surrender, abandon yourself to Him. Maybe just being a good Christian, maybe martyrdom, probably in between.

One can way overdo devotions to the point you get burnt out and then the enemy destroys much of the good God has accomplished through you. Or severely lessens your effectiveness at letting God work through you. That is why one of the enemy's favorite tactics is to get you sleep deprived through unbelievably varied means.

My directors told me I was being called to three main apostolates. How does one know? Prayer, LISTENING, and being nudged by God via various Lives of the Saints, homilies, Breviary readings, scripture, all confirmed this. Teresa of Avila I believe also talks about seeking confirmation from more than one source. I have always found true callings from God He affirms via, for me, homilies, readings of the Bible, Breviary, and LISTENING to Him and my priests, directors. He affirms it three times within a week. Remember this is old hard headed me, but experienced me. We are all different. But we all should seek affirmation, confirmation. And we all should know He does not want us praying non-stop 20 hours a day. Probably eight may be approaching a maximum, with "recreations" a cloistered nun term, or chores, or fun, interspersed.

So what are some good devotions? Oh my there are so many, and many I do not do or only due to a certain extent. Seek guidance and be cautious!

I have personal prayers that, as I read the lives of Saints, God seemed to lean over and say, "Write that one down, and pray it." I have found often after praying that prayer

For a month or a year, fruit came forth and then God said, "Now move on to this prayer." As if I had completed something He wanted for myself or others and now had a new task a new lesson.

So, what are my devotions etc. Well I have several <u>personal prayers</u>. I pray two or three on rising, I shower, and then do my first <u>readings from the Breviary (Divine Office, Office of Readings, Liturgy of the Hours</u>, all these are the same names for the prayers priests, religious and third order seculars pray daily). Then I turn to <u>intercessory prayer</u> and offer up my Mass and or Communion that day for them as well. I have a prayer list where I write down requests. You may find you have hundreds. In that case I advise do what Bernadette and Therese did. Hold them and pray, "Papa, Jesus, Holy Spirit, I pray for all of these. Draw us to yourself and help us as You will." I tried and tired praying for 30-50+ people by name every day, bad idea when you are sick.

I pray the Rosary for the Souls in Purgatory—Saint Gertrude's Prayers. I pray the Divine Mercy Novena for nine days then start over again. Many do. I pray the prayers regarding devotion to the Holy Face as I am a member of the Archconfraternity of the Holy Face in Tours, France. Don't get too impressed it takes bout 10 minutes.

I pray Therese's Chaplet, this is so very soothing to me and such a great grace, and as I pray it I thank God and tell Him I love Him.

And I now pray the 20 decade rosary. I used to say, "O that's impossible unless you have whole days etc." It takes about 30 minutes, and that is with contemplation.

I have a friend who says, "Oh don't do verbal prayer, contemplate." And I have a priest who ordered me to contemplate twice daily for five to sixty minutes for the rest of my life. Not for the weak of heart initially, later . . . too much of a blessing for a little nothing like me. The first weeks you may just sit and try and listen for five to sixty minutes. St. Teresa said this can go on for years. But Oh, it is worth it!

There is an excellent book, by Rt. Rev. Dom Vitalis Lehodey, <u>"The Ways of Mental Prayer."</u> Tan Books and Publishers,

Rockford; 1982. It reviews Vocal, Mental and Mystical Prayer and all the types, I highly recommend it. Remember, to follow the advice of your spiritual director, and Saint and Doctor of the Church, Teresa of Avila, "it is not up to us, God will grant it in His time, surrender to Him", and be honest with yourself.

There are also excellent books on numerous Novenas, and on numerous Rosaries and Chaplets at Catholic bookstores.

One of my very early prayers comes from the Devotion of the Sacred Heart. My wife prays the Seven Sorrows of Mary. And we both monthly pray the Franciscan seven decade Crown Rosary. Daily we pray the prayers attached to Devotion to the Holy Face of Christ independently, and at times together.

So, to summarize there are hundreds of prayers, devotions, rosaries, and chaplets. Use your spiritual director and discernment to learn what God wants you to do; and be careful to not add extras and overdo. Usually 2-3 are the average.

Chapter 6

Discernment

We have talked about this but it bears repeating. Anyone can offer up their sufferings to God, for the poor souls in Purgatory and for the conversion of sinners. It is a very old Catholic tradition and lends value and purpose to our suffering.

But, is God asking you to be a <u>victim</u> of suffering? **This is more rare**. Is he asking you to become like His Son one who takes on suffering for the salvation and redemption of His children. This takes discernment. I believe that for most it comes as a surprise, they were not thinking about it. Many may deny this tugging on the heart for a time. God is a gentleman, He will very quietly, patiently ask you, "Will you do this for me? He will await your answer. He can be very persistent. Your answer may be "Yes." And you may find He was only asking to see if you loved Him enough to say yes. You may deny you are hearing Him for a long time. I did, Jonah did. But God is patient and persistent. He will keep asking. You may say "No".

No, to the one who loves you most and consistently, regardless of your screw ups. No, to being able to help Him, to help the one who did the same for you. No, to a dramatically greater knowledge and participation in His love. Will He hate you? I don't think so, He gave you free will. Will He be disappointed? He probably knew what your answer would be all along and asked it to get you to thinking about your life and how you are living it, to give you a chance for more; more of His love, more intense living of this life, more in the next life.

Am I really hearing God, or am I being deceived by the enemy, or am I going nuts? These are pretty much your three possibilities. I knew I was not worthy so assumed insanity. But I knew enough about my faith to see it could be God and so investigate, and that is what you will want to do. Investigate and find the source. The best way is through experienced good spiritual directors. Again, usually there will be a Nun or priest or secular third order who knows of someone, they themselves go to or have referred others to successfully.

Read <u>St. Teresa of Avila</u>, St. John of the Cross and perhaps St. Bonaventure. All have excellent writings on discernment. Though all three are doctors of the Church and widely and for centuries accepted as THE experts, the first two are most commonly recommended.

Pray, ask God. Beg Him to not allow you to be led astray. Mean it. Know yourself, are you prideful, prone to jump to conclusions? If so you really need a good, experienced spiritual director, and to LISTEN!

LISTEN. You can't get the answer if you don't listen. Listen to: 1) God 2) Teresa, John, Catherine of Siena 3) your priest spiritual director.

How do you know if it's God talking. He is usually quiet, remember Ezekiel? He heard God not in the thunder, or earthquake, not in the violent wind, but in the soft whispering breeze. God is quiet, a gentleman, a Father. He never lies. He loves to be questioned for it shows you care and are discerning. So question Him. Ask for more affirmation/confirmation from the above, from homilies, scripture etc. Remember if it is of God usually you will have unrest/fear then peace. The enemy will usually leave you with a deceitful peace that turns into unrest as the Holy Spirit tries to warn you.

Chapter 7

The Value of Spiritual Directors

I think we have discussed this over and over. St. Teresa certainly does. A bad spiritual director can really slow you down, lead you astray, or at least stall your growth. Also, remember God loves those who are obedient. Many saints were given bad advice to test them and God was so proud when they told Him what they were to do and were obedient. You see they talk everything over with God, and listen to His answer.

A good spiritual director will ask you many questions to learn about you and what you think is going on and why. He will have been through it before so can tell what is going on and advise you. He will be honest. He will warn you about the enemy, about how he will use your weak areas to cause you to fall and become discouraged. He will encourage you to: attend Mass daily, go to confession weekly or monthly depending on your parish and how able they are to meet the needs of the parish regarding confession.

He will encourage you to read St. Teresa and later St. John of the Cross and other Saints and other spiritual reading.

He will encourage you to grow in your relationship with Mary and pray the rosary. He may well encourage you to read about the various kinds of prayer and to attempt to contemplate even though you may not be successful in this immediately. He may well encourage you to do an examination of your conscience every night before bed.

Padre Pio did this, it was his routine counseling to others seeking to grow in their love of God. My spiritual directors went over these things. Be prepared to fall ever more deeply in love with Christ, ever more pure. If you do not notice you are growing in the virtues, something is wrong. And be prepared to grow in your devotion to the poor souls in Purgatory.

If you need prayer seek out cloistered nuns, their love for God and therefore their effectiveness at prayer is awesome. I have two groups of Franciscan Poor Clare Nuns, one in Illinois and one in Cincinnati; and two of Carmelite Discalced Nuns One in Pennsylvania and one in Lisieux France, I turn to.

I was told I would be shocked to know how many Saints were in my Church by my director; that I was not alone in my quest to seek, love and obey God more. So, you are not alone, but in five years I have only found one or two other mystically "blessed" person(s) who would share with me about it.

Oh, and he will probably tell you to not talk to anyone about how God is dealing with you except your director or confessor; and urge you to keep a journal of your experiences. He may advise you have these journals given to the Church for examination after your death.

Conclusion

Well, I hope I have been of some help. I was just sitting here doing Christmas Cards when God spoke to me about this. Actually I was also talking with Him about my recent worsening of my illness and surrendering myself to Him, and reflecting on my journey and all His help and love. So I guess you were on His mind and He figured I would make a handy secretary to type this up. He has me write some really great stuff and I always am amazed because I know it did not come from me. At least not just me, alone, I would not have done this, and could not have, on my own.

God bless you in your journey, see you at the end.

PS:

If you are married I think it's good to not allow your prayer life to interfere with your spending time with your family or just being available to them. Mine know if they catch me praying to feel very free to interrupt. I generally on my wife's days off get up at 0400, ouch (remember true love) and can get much done way ahead of time. Or I can continue while she cooks, or is out running errands or working on a project of her own, or after she goes to bed. Isn't that tiring up from 0400 to midnight? Yes, but I respect my needs and nap the next day and only do this a few times a week if absolutely necessary. What about staying with family over holidays etc. I work this the same way. By the way I find after about 3 days I get grumpy. Why? I have less time alone with Christ. I think it's because I'm not mature enough yet, I need to increase my praising Him and telling Him I love Him when I am interacting with others. I do my spiritual reading in that little special office (the bathroom) many times.

ADDENDUM:

I finished this book around May of 2010. Then in September I read a book by Therese's closest novice, Marie of the Trinity (during the last years of her life half her face was a horrible wound from lupus), and I quote some beautiful quotes in this book, Therese of Lisieux and Marie of the Trinity by Pierre Descouvemont, St. Paul Press.

"The Christian who suffers knows he is not alone. He is freed forever from the pain of suffering "for nothing": his wounds are a source of grace for all mankind.

> "This word of the prophet: 'The Lord wounds only to heal' (Hosea 6:1), helps me a lot when I think of my lupus. Yes, all our wounds—physical or moral—united with those of Jesus, serve to heal souls. What grace to be thus associated with redemption!"

In His mercy the Lord was going ahead of His spouse in the trial she will undergo later on. How true is this good Theresian doctrine, coming straight from John of the Cross: God always makes us desire what He will one day give to us. In confiding to Fr. Marie-Bernard on July 21, 1941, that the progress of her illness permitted her to eat only with great difficulty, the sick nun added:

> "God gives me the grace not to be apprehensive about the future. I abandon myself to Him like a child to the best of fathers who acts for the best. My great consolation is to regard the sorrowful face of Jesus and ascertain some traits of resemblance with it. Sr. Therese of the Child Jesus often loved to remind me of these words of Isaiah: "He is without beauty and renown, He has nothing to attract the eye and we have despised Him," etc. (Is 52:2-3). I have been wondering about her insistence of always coming back to this same subject. Now I truly believe that God inspired her in order to tell me these things that would do me so much good later on."

The presence of Therese was sometimes granted to Marie by a delicious fragrance that all of a sudden invaded the place she found herself in.

> "I almost regret having told you this. I'm afraid that you might think Therese loves you less because you haven't received all these favors, but it's completely to the contrary! I'm quit convinced, in fact, that if I had been stronger, less beaten down, Therese would never have done that and it is more of a consternation to me to see that my imperfection almost forces her to grant me this favor. These kinds of graces are never granted on earth as a reward for virtue but only as an encouragement. Here below, the reward for virtue, the proof of God's contentment with us, is trial, temptations, sufferings of all kinds . . . Ah! How you deceive yourself to want to believe otherwise."

> "No, Therese doesn't spare her true friends, she rather allows them to be engraved in the image of Jesus."

Being with Therese, the novice had particularly understood that joy is one of the first—fruits of the Spirit, as the apostle Paul says (Gal 5:22). Allegremente! (joyously, merrily) Philip Neri liked to repeat, and we know the joyful—even playful—atmosphere which characterized the meetings of his disciples in the oratory. This was the atmosphere Therese wanted to see reigning in the Novitiate entrusted to her. Like her spiritual mother, Teresa of Avila, she was convinced that far from impeding union with God, Such an ambience would favor it.

In line with the spiritual tradition, Therese spotted the importance of the warfare that needs to be carried out against the disease that the ancients denounced under the name of apathy. Already in the second century the Shepherd of Hermas had denounced the bad effects of this harmful sadness: "Every joyful person acts well, thinks right and tramples sadness underfoot. The sad person to the contrary, always acts badly by saddening the Holy Spirit who is given to mankind as joy; second, he commits an impiety in not praying to the Lord, because the prayer of a sad person doesn't have the strength to mount up to the altar of God. Sadness mixed with prayer prevents it from rising, like vinegar mixed with wine takes away its taste. Purify your heart of harmful sadness, then, and you will live for God."

For Therese, joy was above all one of the privileged ways of expressing her love to God. It was one very simple way for us to tell Him how much we appreciate His infinite tenderness and mercy and that we don't blame Him for the sufferings whose presence He permits in our lives as pilgrims.

I agree, joy shows God how much we rejoice in His loving us, and how we love Him!

PPS:

St. Rose's of Viterbo, a young 18 year old secular Franciscan's, dying words to her parents were: "I die with joy, for I desire to be united to my God. Live so as not to fear death. For those who live well (spiritually) in the world, death is not frightening, but sweet and precious."

DEATH & DYING THE JOURNEY PART II.

Please note: This first section of Part II. is the actual lecture I gave to doctors, nurses, aides and family care givers for 25 years at their request. It is to the point, and covers serious, emotional information. It may be too much for some people, unless you really feel a need to know and so better help the dying.

OBJECTIVES: Attendees will be able to:

- Identify their own feelings associated with caring for the dying.
- Explore their personal feelings and questions associated with death and the loss of loved ones and understand these feelings in patients and family.
- Identify the stages of dying and comfort measures appropriate to these symptoms.
- List the stages of grieving and how to help patients and families through these.
- Recognize the needs of the patient, family, and other heath care providers.
- Identify rituals and beliefs associated with death in various cultures.
- Learn from St. Therese of Lisieux how one can experience this journey.
- Learn also from St. Paul, St. Bonaventure of Potenza & others how to "finish the race".

The Big Questions of My Life—everyone should fill one of these out.

- Name:_____ Date: _____
- I will give a copy of this to:_____

- 1. What is the purpose of my life?
- 2. Is there a God?
- 3. Is there something more than this life? Something after this life?
- The Big Questions of My Life—Continued
- 4. What will happen to me when I die?
- 5. What happens to those I love when they die?
- 6. Will I see them again?
- 7. Will I die alone?
- 8. This is the funeral I want:
- Music:
- Readings:
- Location of Ceremonies:
- What I want done with my body:
- What I want on my tombstone:

My Background:

I have worked with the dying and their loved ones and care givers since 1970. I have experienced the anxiety of not knowing what to say or do, the guilt of wondering did I do every thing I could have, should have. I have experienced the <u>loss</u> of these "friends". I have been guided by my mentor and role model, and wife, Dolores Gillen, to ask myself the big questions of life so that by facing my own mortality, and my own feelings, I could learn to cope with death and loss of myself and loved ones. I could be comfortable with death and dying and so be able to sit down with those doing it and be someone who could listen and help them through this last leg of life's journey.

My Experience:

- Nurses aide 1970-78, and Diener-one who assists with autopsies, for me 900,
- RN 1978-80 Coronary and Intensive Care,—1980—current nurse specialist in wounds and ostomies majority of my patients had Coronary Artery Disease, chronic lung disease, Renal disease, diabetes or cancer, and many were dying. I was there to hold hands of the dying, and then support the family.
- 1970-1997 33 Codes, cardiac resuscitation attempts, majority successful.
- <u>Personal Losses</u>: Lost my Father-in-law COPD 1979, Father MI 1993, Mother with her 2nd cancer 2002, Nephew at 30, 1993 melanoma, friend at 20, 2007 car accident, I nearly lost my daughter to leukemia 13-16, 1995-1998. She beat it! I had Pre-melanoma of my R eye 1998. So I have lost people I love to death, & had near brushes with it with myself and others.

And I have talked to and listened to my God and my dear friend, Therese.

Personal History of Death.—every one should fill out one of these.

- 1. The first death I remember was the death of:
- 2. I was age:
- 3. I remember the feelings of:
- 4. The first funeral I was ever at was:
- 5. I was age:
- 6. The one thing I remember most was:
- 7. My most recent loss was:
- 8. I cope with this loss by:
- 9. The most difficult death for me was:
- 10. It was difficult because:
- 11. Of all the people in my life now living, the most difficult death for me would be:
- 12. It would be most difficult because:
- 13. My primary style of coping with loss is:
- 14. I know my own grief is resolved when:
- 15. It is appropriate to share my own experiences of grief with another when:
- From: J.W. Worden, "Grief Counseling and Grief Therapy: A handbook for the Mental Health Practitioner" (2nd Edition). New York, NY: Springer Press, 199".

The Process of Dying

This is a rough outline of the stages of death and symptoms.

- Patients may groan but this is seldom due to pain. It may be an attempt to talk. Remember the if patient needs pain relief, addiction is NOT an issue when one is terminal, that is dying within say 6 months.
- Even should they become unresponsive pain medicine should not be stopped as the pain will return, but the pain medicine may be reduced to ¼ the prior dose if needed.
- Patients become weaker, they become uninterested in food or drink, they are not rejecting family, simply drawing away, thinking, resting. They may have problems swallowing and now we believe that food and drink may result in edema, nausea and increased pain from tumor growth. Endorphins may be released that relieve pain etc. from lack of food and water.
- Bowels and kidneys function less which may be a blessing to the patient, a simple chux pad changed as needed avoids having to jostle them around, or placing them on a bed pan etc.
- Respirations will vary with periods of shallow breathing and lack of breathing. Rattling noises may occur and can be lessened by position changes. These occur 2-3 days prior to death. Patients may gasp for breath, oxygen usually will not help but morphine and a fan blowing on their face can.
- the heart rate may increase with faster breathing. Morphine reduces oxygen consumption and relieves anxiety and breathlessness and will lower the heart rate.
- Patients may become restless due to pain, electrolyte imbalance, dehydration, or opiate metabolites. Hydration may help. Sedatives such as Haldol may help. They may have a full bladder that we can help them empty. We can help with these. They may just need reassurance they

are not alone, touch and talking to them may be the best answer.

- As they proceed on their journey they <u>may</u> become less responsive and even comatose around 6 hours prior to death.
- As they become dehydrated the heart rate increases, slowly the blood pressure drops, and then the heart rate decreases.
- The skin becomes cold due to slowing metabolism and decreased intake and activity and circulation. They don't usually feel cold and piling on blankets may be uncomfortable to the patient.
- Mottling occurs over the knees, soles of feet, bony prominences and on lower body parts usually around 5 hours prior to death.
- Bright light hurts their eyes, but a dim light helps them feel less alone.
- Listen, talk briefly with them, touch them.

The Stages of Grieving

Elizabeth Kubler-Ross was the first person to really look at grieving and to try and put it into stages we could recognize and help others go through. More recently some lump these into 3 stages. Please note stages can recur, occur out of order, etc. I still like this way of looking at things.

Kubler-Ross 5 Stages of Grieving
Denial: "It can't be."
Anger: "Why me."
Bargaining: "I'll change if I only . . ."
Depression "I don't care anymore."
Acceptance: "I'm ready."

Newer categories:
- Numbness: Shock disbelief, social isolation, running on auto-pilot

- Disorganization: confusion, aimless, can't think, feelings of loss, helplessness
- Reorganization: getting back into the game of life

There are also classifications of: Normal Grief and of other variations encountered

Anticipatory Grief: Grieving before the event occurs

Children's Grief: Children experience loss in different ways and have different coping needs based on their stage of development.

Complicated Grief:

Usually occurs in people regarding unusual death i.e. sudden, unexpected, traumatic; or with a history of poor coping or mental health issues. It is also associated with lack of support systems, and a lack of spiritual beliefs.

Delayed: Normal grief postponed by circumstances.

Chronic: Grief continues beyond normal 1-2 years.

Exaggerated: Abnormal behaviors such as suicide occurs.

Masked: Person unaware how grief is impairing functioning.

Disenfranchised: Grief when relationship carries a social stigma i.e., death of a lover who is married to another, gay, ex-spouse, AIDs pt.

What can we do?

Sometimes on our journey through life we get lost. Some parts go faster, others slower. How can we help each other?

Find out where they are in their journey. Go to their room. Sit down-it tells them and us we have time to care for them. Spend time with them. Ask, "How are you doing with all of this?" It shows them they are not alone, and it gives them permission to work out their own thoughts and questions about life's big mysteries.

There maybe times that denial is just too hard. That keeping "it" a secret is too much work. Then it is time we help them to drop the mask, and tell people what is going on. This time came for my daughter. We let her stay home from school and her teacher shared the news with all her classmates. What a burden was lifted.

There will be times they feel like they are going crazy. This is normal. Again, we need to take time to be with them and give them permission to vent, and tell them it's normal.

What do we say?—"I don't know what to say, what if I say the wrong thing?"

"I'm sorry you are going through this."

"This must be hard."

"It's okay to feel the way you do."

"I can bring dinner over on Tuesday or Thursday, which is best for you?"

"Working through this takes time, try and be patient with yourself."

"You will never forget_____will you?"

"_____meant a lot to you. Tell me about them."

"Its not easy, what will you miss the most?"

All of these are excellent and time proven.

Remember: being silent and listening and a gentle touch go a long way.

The Patient's Needs & the Needs of Others

I have been involved in helping others deal with death & dying since around 1970. Since 1997 I have been researching it and sad to say based on 2002-05 information I have to conclude that American's are not facing death with less fear. They are not achieving good deaths. My experiences into 2010-11 haven't changed this opinion.

They feel that we as providers of health care are not well prepared and are not meeting their needs. What do they need?

They need answers. They need to know when medical care is no longer effective and may even adversely effect quality of life. They want doctors to talk about the medical outlook, comfort care, palliative care, hospice—<u>early on</u>. They need us to give them choices and a sense of control.

They want to know what community resources are available to help them and their families. Our medical social workers are THE people who make this do-able, and mean so very much to us.

They need us to help clarify priorities, and promote informed choices. Having made their decisions they need us to respect their wishes and opinions and help them cope.

They need us to be there for them. To just have time to *listen* to their end-of-life concerns. Give them permission to ask questions and to talk.

The Patient's Needs

They want to be cared for by people who are knowledgeable and compassionate, and who maintain a sense of hope & optimism. Not false hope, maybe just a good day.

They and their families fear they will be in pain. This is a major concern. Reassure them we will work with them and provide comfort. We will respond with the right medicine and interventions at the right dose routinely. Though we fear them becoming addicted, of giving them the "last shot" that sends them over the edge, we will conquer these feelings because they have no place in the care of the dying.

Another major fear is of dying alone. Help them know this by being there for them, stopping in, spending time, never being in a hurry to leave, take a minute & fluff a pillow,

Understand they feel they are a burden. Help them see we are happy to be a part of it all. We all see it as a privilege. One of my best comments to a patient feeling this was, "You are a burden." They looked wide eyed, I said, "Do you know how heavy a gold bar is?" They nodded yes. I said, "Well that gold, to carry it is a real burden, but would anyone turn a gold bar down? You are like that, a <u>very</u> <u>precious</u> burden."

I also told a patient, "You may be losing your leg or breast but we, me and your family we love all of you we don't care if a piece or two are missing, we want all that's left."

Preserve their dignity. See them as a human being, one that matters.

Moving closer & maintaining eye contact for most shows we care. Some cultures see this as disrespect, so be sensitive, be close, & look them in the eye, if it doesn't offend.

Listen and talk to them, be aware that hearing is the last to go.

Help them mend relationships early, and accomplish life tasks, get spiritual care.

Help them find and maintain support systems be it family, friends, church, clubs, etc. All provide individuals to lighten the load.

People are afraid to talk about death and dying. They want to help but don't know what to do. Take time to discern this. To help them be comfortable and play whatever part they are comfortable with.

Don't forget children and making them a part of this loving team. Prepare them for this. Answer their questions, help them know this is just a part of life, no one did anything wrong. In doing this we make their life and deaths easier as they grow older.

They need us to meet their spiritual needs. Patients & families are telling us we are failing in this area. The need may just be for us to listen. It may be for us to offer to call their church, or the chaplain. Hospitals in an effort to comply with HIPPA regulations are not notifying ministers of patient's admission. This robs them of a support system. Maybe they are not from this area, or haven't been able to get to church in a while, offer to help them locate a local caring minister. Respect their culture and needs.

When? "When will I die, how much time do I have left?" Many patients will ask this if they perceive you care, and are a good listener. My response was, "I don't know, really no one knows but God. Many doctors are good guessers so if your Dr. told you that you have six weeks, that's probably close. But think of this. The day you are born you start to die. The day you die until the minute of your death you are living. So all our lives we are both living and dying at the same time. Which do you want to focus your last six weeks on, living or dying?"

The Family's Needs

Help them understand the illness and how it will affect the patient, what to expect, and how to deal with these issues and basic care needs.

Educate them regarding resources available.

Remember they are losing a loved one. There may be an injured relationship that needs healing. There may be guilt, or jealousy. There always is anxiety, and fear of failing the pt. and other family.

In general it appears that patients and family prefer that the patient dies at home. It isn't always possible and doesn't happen every time. But in some ways it is easier on them and they are able to better relax.

They want doctors to take the lead and talk early on about end-of-life issues. They need us to be truthful.

They want nurses to help the health team, patient and families to communicate with each other.

They are afraid. They need us to understand. They want to help, to do things for the patient but are afraid and need to know how. Make them comfortable, but don't expect them to do all the baths etc. They are not employees they are family.

They need direct honest communication and updates and our support.

They need us to provide opportunities to negotiate care plans, and make changes as time goes on and situations change. Respect their wishes and opinions.

Help them cope. Encourage them to express their feelings and concerns. Be available to listen. Demonstrate caring. Use touch as needed. Coming closer and look them in the eye usually is seen as signs of caring and acceptance but some cultures avoid this, be sensitive.

Try to be accepting and tolerant. They are going through one of life's biggest challenges, losing a loved one. We're not judges, we're fellow travelers on the same road.

Show them their loved one is important to you too. Treat the patient with respect, gentleness and sensitivity.

Help them find and maintain support systems-family, friends, church, clubs, chaplain etc.

Be aware they might only need your willingness to listen and some respite. Offer concrete help . . . "Why don't you grab a cup of coffee and take a break, I'll stay with your mother."

Just like all of us, families need thanks and praise. Sometimes patients and spouses are too overwhelmed to think to express gratitude. So I take the time to look them in the eye and say . . . "Thanks for being such a great son and caring for your father so well. I know it must be hard for you at times. You are a true blessing to them." Then be ready for the tears. They are appreciated but too often don't hear anyone say it. This may be the memory that outlasts all others.

As the time draws near so many feelings well up: fear, guilt, anger, anxiety, peace, relief even joy. Do they need other family called? Do they need a minister? Respect the moment, respect their close circle, but don't abandon them at this time.

Don't rush away to do paperwork, to notify. Get someone else to do it if possible. You who know them, stay with them a while. Then when it's time ask the family if they want to be alone with the patient and respect that wish.

The best response is, "I'm sorry for your loss."

Calling the funeral home is often best done now helping them make the call from the room. Show your caring, use touch as appropriate.

Finally help them find a bereavement group to plug into for healing.

<u>Quotes from famous patients as they died</u>:

"Beautiful!" — Elizabeth Barrett Browning, writer, died June 28, 1861

"It is very beautiful over there." — Thomas Edison, inventor, died October 18, 1931

"I've never felt better." — Douglas Fairbanks, actor, died December 12, 1939

"Let us cross over the river and sit in the shade of the trees." — General Thomas Stonewall Jackson died 1863

"I die hard but am not afraid to go." — George Washington. December 14, 1799

"O! . . . my God . . . I love Thee . . . Therese of Lisieux 1897

"It is so very beautiful, I wish you could see it too." — A Minister (my patient) 1978

"O no! stop! Get off of me." wailed & gnashed teeth (Had been filled with guilt and hate and refused religion.) Another of my patients same day in 1978.

The Health Care Providers Needs (Physicians, Nurses, Techs, family care givers

As health care providers most of us come to the hospital with very little experience with death and dying, and for some what little they find is negative. We are just people too with the same fears and anxieties. But unlike our patients we will likely face death many more times. We will lose perhaps hundreds of patients and family.

I believe to be a good health care provider you must care about the patient. They must matter to you. If you care they will sense this and trust you enough to work with you in achieving the health attainable by them. If you care your relationship with them will grow and involve their loved ones, and like it or not, they become family to you. This is the great reward that is ours. It also means however that we will experience the loss of more people in our lives. If we don't learn how to handle these losses we will be destroyed.

Health care providers face stress and anxiety from two sources. 1) The fear of death to include our own. 2) Not knowing what to do, not feeling prepared. Hopefully we have addressed both of these and have less anxiety and feel better prepared. But what about our colleagues, all those around us, to include the doctors?

Recognize their hurts and needs as well. We are all the same, people, all experiencing losses and striving to cope.

We need to help each other, realize that death is not a failure. It is a natural, normal part of life. The goal is not always cure. The goal is striving to obtain the best quality life and death possible. Ira Byock MD said in reflecting on his father's death, "When the human dimension of dying is nurtured, for many the transition from life can become as profound, intimate and precious as the miracle of birth." I, a nurse of 40 years agree.

We are all patients, we are all health care providers to each other. Sometimes the patient becomes the teacher, & even physician to you.

Peers need our touch, our time, and our asking, "How are you feeling?"

42

We need to help each other find support systems. Community, family, church, clubs, friends. Be part of their support system, invite them to become part of yours.

Taking care of the dying is hard work. Let each other know you understand, "This must be hard for you." and that you appreciate them, "Thanks for all you're doing for the patient and their family. It means a lot." Everyone needs thanks and praise.

Too many deaths, too many losses unresolved leads to burnout and loss of peers to drugs, illness, suicide and leaving a caring profession forever.

One of the best oncologists I have ever known quit after one death too many and became a pharmaceutical rep. Two heart doctors took a leave of absence when an 18 year old died after reconstructive surgery. I found two surgeons crying in a stairwell over the death of an elderly man who they had cared for all their practice lives. The loss is real, the pain is real, the cure is talking. We need to find someone to talk to and vent, a co-worker, a peer, the chaplain, a minister, our God, our family.

We need to pour out our feelings so healing can begin. To reflect and see death really is just a normal part of living. A chance to live, love and move on taking with us the good memories of peace and pain free passing and the help we did render. Remember Golden Pond with Katherine Hepburn and Henry Fonda? Norman talks about death and Ethel is in denial. After Norman almost dies Ethel tells him, "I could actually see you in the casket and I didn't like it, it was cold." Norman says "And now what?" and she replies, "Well its not so bad, natural, warm, even comforting, like an old friend."

We all need someone to talk to. Please do. If you have no one handy talk to me. I'm not a priest, I'm not a mental health person, I'm just Pat a fellow traveler on life's journey.

Cultural Aspects of Dying as of 2008

America is becoming more culturally diversified, therefore we need to be able to look through end-of-life care through different eyes so we are not prejudiced and allow false concepts and biases to detract from our care.

Did you know women are perceived to not need opiates? No basis in fact. That the elderly see pain as expected so don't mention it? That they have a hard time relating to we younger providers as they are used to having doctors older than they are. That children are often under-medicated because of our fears of addicting them, and that parents may deny they have pain because they are trying to deny their illness.

Various ethnic groups look at things differently. Hispanics/ Latinos and Chinese and Native Americans avoid eye contact out of respect. Elders are usually respected and the family often makes the patient's decisions with the patient becoming passive in their care. Patients are more stoic and deny pain.

Hispanics feel it is bad luck to die in a hospital, the soul will get lost. Chinese patients feel dying at home is bad luck.

Native Americans feel associating with the dying is bad luck so patients may prefer hospitals as family may avoid them. Many groups want to hide the terminal diagnosis from the patient.

Various religions have different rituals and preferences regarding dying.

Catholics may request a priest to provide the anointing of the sick—no longer for dying only but for getting well; confession and communion.

Orthodox believers may request anointing as well and also have confession and communion, memorial feast is held about 40 days after death, in Catholics this is held one year later, both help families cope.

Protestants may request prayers, and some anoint.

Seven Day Adventists don't believe in blood transfusions.

Jews and Muslims avoid any form of pork and Muslims all alcohol. Beef, mutton & poultry must be prepared in a special way. Both may prefer vegetarian diets.

Muslims do not like to discuss death. Cousins and Uncles usually are the contact persons who determine what the pt. is told. Patients may chose to face Mecca and have their head elevated. Only same sex Muslims may touch the body, and grief may be expressed by slapping.

Jews want everything done to prolong life. A dying person should never be left alone and a Rabbi's presence is desired. After death the body is placed on the floor, covered with a sheet, with the feet towards the door and a candle at the head. IF they die at home on a Sabbath, the body cannot be moved until the next day.

Hindus also prefer a vegetarian diet. Death is accepted and a priest will assist. Rituals include tying a red thread around the wrist or neck and sprinkling them with water from the Ganges River, a basil leaf may be placed on the tongue. After death the body is not washed and the thread not removed.

Buddhists are also vegetarians and believe in reincarnation. Patients should be asked about special diet needs. A shrine of Buddha may be placed in the room and time for meditation is important and should be respected. They want to have a clear mind and so medications may be refused. Buddhists accept death and a monk may recite prayers at death for an hour.

African Americans may fear pain medications and shortness of breath at the end of life. Usually the spouse and elders address care decisions. Church is seen as a strong support system and members like family.

Since it is the patient who is dying and the family who are going through loss, we need to be aware of these cultural factors and assess what their beliefs and desires are so we may respect and help them.

Resources:

(These are from when I gave this lecture in 2008 at Wright-Patterson, due an internet search and learn what's available. Another excellent source is the local Hospice.)

Living with Loss Support Group Wright-Patterson
Hospital Chaplains Services 257-8900 or Medical Social Work 257-6429

Survivors of Suicide, SOS
Miami Valley Hospital 1-800-320-4357

Resolve Through Sharing RTS Hospital Birthing Center Wright-Patterson
Medical Social Work 257-6429

Oak Tree Corner—Children's Grief Services
285-0199

Death & Heaven St. Therese of Lisieux

When we start on a journey it is comforting to have a road map or at least talk with someone who has been there. The following are quotes I thought might help.

"It's not death that will come in search of me, it's God. Death isn't some phantom, some horrible spectre as revealed in some picture (the grim reaper). Death is the separation of the soul from the body and that is all it is."

"I don't know when I shall die. I no longer have any confidence in this illness. I will not be sure of success until I find myself in God's arms."

"All is vanity, worthless, except loving God."

"Now I have no desire left, unless it be to love Jesus even to folly! It is love that draws me."

"From childhood I felt that one day I should be free from this land of darkness. I believed it, not only because I had been told so by others, but my heart's most secret and deepest longings assured me that there was in store for me another and more beautiful country—an abiding dwelling place. I was like Christopher Columbus who anticipated the discovery of a new world."

"Be comforted, all passes away. Our life of yesterday is spent; death too will come and go, then we shall rejoice in life, true life, for countless ages for evermore."

"The greatest honor God can bestow upon a soul is not to give it great things but to ask of it great things."

"I am not dying, I am entering into Life . . ." St. Therese

"What is this mysterious separation of the souls from the body? It's my first experience of this, but I abandon myself to God."

She loved God so much she wanted to be with Him, she asked her prioress permission to die and was denied this. She confided to a friend, "When the Thief approaches, the community will yell 'Thief, Thief!' but I will wave my hands and say, 'Here, here.'"

Therese had a new way of looking at things, a Gospel way, a "little way". She believed she could not climb the steep stairs of perfection. But would instead admit her littleness and unworthiness and ask forgiveness when she fell. She knew God understands we are weak and toddlers spiritually. So she believed she could stand at the bottom of the steep stairs and raise her arms and her God, "Papa" would bend down and lift her up and embrace her.

"With me prayer is simply an uplifting of the heart; a glance towards heaven; a cry of gratitude and love, uttered equally in sorrow and in joy. In a word it is something noble, supernatural, which expands my soul and unites it to God."

She was once found crying in her cell. When asked why she said, "I was saying the Our Father, O! to be able to call Him that!"

"I realized that Heaven does exist, and that this Heaven is peopled with souls who cherish me as their child, and this impression still remains with me."

"I thirst after Heaven, that blessed abode where our love for Jesus will be without bounds. True, we must pass through suffering and tears to reach that home, but I wish to suffer all that my Beloved is pleased to send me; I wish to let Him do as He wills with his little one."

"It is not death that will come to fetch me, it is the good God. Death is no phantom, no horrible spectre, as represented in pictures. In the Catechism it is stated that death is the separation of soul and body, that is all! Well, I am not afraid of a separation which will unit me to the good God forever." Counsels and Reminiscences

One day she said to Mother Prioress: "Mother, I beseech you, give me permission to die . . .

Let me offer my life for . . ." mentioning the intention. And this permission being refused:

"Very well," she resumed, "I know that at this moment the good God so much desires *a littlebunch of grapes* which no one wishes to present to Him, that He will certainly be forced to come and steal it . . . I ask nothing, for that would be to depart from my way of abandonment, I merely beg the Blessed Virgin Mary to recall to her Jesus the blessed title of *Thief* which He gives Himself in the Holy Gospel, so that He may not forget to come and steal me away." Story of a Soul Ch 12

"Will the Divine Thief be coming soon to steal His little bunch of grapes?" Someone asked.

I see Him afar off, and I take good care not to cry out, "Stop Thief!" On the contrary I call Him saying: "This way! This way!"

"Ah! If the Divine Master would permit those who are about to leave for His love but one glimpse of the glory in store, and the vast retinue of souls that will escort you to Heaven, already you would be repaid for the great sacrifice that is at hand." *("Eye has not seen nor ear heard, nor has the mind of man conceived what God has prepared for those who love Him.")*

"What mysteries will yet be unveiled to us? I have often thought that perhaps I owe all the graces with which I am laden, to some little soul whom I shall only know in Heaven.

It is God's will that in this world souls shall dispense to each other, by prayer, the treasures of Heaven, in order that when they reach their Everlasting Home they may love one another with grateful hearts, and with an affection far in excess of that which reigns in the most perfect family on earth."

Her last words, "O I love You. O! . . . My God . . . I love You so!"

From Divine Intimacy by Father Gabriel of Mary Magdalen OCD

"O Lord, the road of trials is the way by which You lead those You love, and the more You Love them, the more trials You send them, since You admit to Your friendship only souls that love the Cross . . . If You asked me whether I should prefer to endure all the trials in the world up to the end of time, and afterwards to gain a little more glory, or to have no trials and to obtain one degree less of glory, I should answer that I would most gladly accept all the trials in exchange for a little more fruition in the understanding of Your wonders, for I see that the more we know You, the more we love and glorify You.

"No, I do not wish to make anything of passing troubles, when it is a question of procuring some glory for You who suffered so much for us."

"If I want to know, O my God, how You act towards those who beg You from the bottom of Their heart to accomplish Your will in them, I have only to ask Your glorious Son, who addressed the same prayer to You in the Garden of Olives . . . You fulfilled this wish in Him by giving Him up to all kinds of sorrows, insults, and persecutions, leaving Him finally to die on the Cross. This is what You gave the one who loved You above all others. As long as we are in this world, these are Your gifts. You proportion them according to Your love for us; You give more to those You love more, and less to those You love less. You also give in accordance to the courage You find in each of us, and according to our love for You, for if we love You much, we shall be able to suffer much for You; whereas if we love you only a little, we will suffer little." St. Teresa of Avila

O my God, dilate my poor heart and make it endure much for love of You. I shall willingly accept suffering, in order to prove to You the reality of my love.

WHY?

There is an old Catholic Tradition that I have come to embrace and love. It may be used by anyone, but especially by those who are suffering and dying, and those who are seeing a loved one suffer and die. Our parents used to say, "Offer up" your suffering for others, for the souls in purgatory and that sinners may have their hearts and minds opened to God's love.

Did not Jesus suffer and die for our sins and those in purgatory? Did not Mary suffer greatly in seeing her Son suffer and die?

So when we suffer the physical pain of suffering; when we suffer the emotional pain of losing a loved one or seeing that one suffer. When we suffer the mental pain of what will happen next to me, to those I love; when we suffer the spiritual pain of becoming angry or paranoid over little things. We can offer all these pains up for the release of the poor souls from purgatory into heaven and that sinners may have their hearts and minds opened to God's love.

When my daughter Kathy was undergoing chemotherapy and suffering she looked at me one day and said, "You know what makes all this worth it? It's knowing that somehow by going through this I am helping others." Indeed this can be a tremendous source of strength and comfort. Knowing our suffering does not have to be in vain and can be a real help to others. <u>And, not just help them for a time but to help give them eternal life, and God their eternal love.</u>

Therese entered Carmel to pray and suffer for sinners, poor souls and priests. She often expressed the hope she could be a martyr. I'll be honest years ago I thought martyrdom was silly. Why, I would fight to defend my faith, not sacrifice myself. But then one day I realized that what better reason to die than to die for others. Not for money by working overtime 20 years, not just for country, but for people, individuals, AND . . . for THE one I love the most.

Death—Therese & Marie of the Trinity

<u>From: "What I Will Soon See For the First Time." from the Poems of Therese</u>:

"Oh! What a moment! What inexpressible happiness,
When I will hear the sweet sound of Your voice,
When I will see in Your adorable Face,
Divine brilliance for the first time! . . .

In heaven, always intoxicated with tenderness,
I will love You without measure and without laws
And my happiness will seem to me endless
As new as the first time!"

<u>Therese of Lisieux and Marie of the Trinity</u> by Pierre Descouvemont, St. Paul Press.

"The Christian who suffers knows he is not alone. He is freed forever from the pain of suffering "for nothing": his wounds are a source of grace for all mankind. "This word of the prophet: 'The Lord wounds only to heal' (Hosea 6:1), helps me a lot when I think of my lupus. Yes, all our wounds—physical or moral—united with those of Jesus, serve to heal souls. What grace to be thus associated with redemption!"

"No, Therese doesn't spare her true friends, she rather allows them to be engraved in the image of Jesus."

References of Death & Dying:

From lectures from 2005-2008 to health Care providers. In 1980 or so I began giving lectures at churches who contacted me on death & dying and these were from family care givers mostly who were afraid because of what they didn't know. Also I did a huge research project on how to help patient, family and healthcare providers cope and these were some of the research articles.

Babcock E. Caring at the Twilight of Life. On the Job Issue. www. Yanton.net; Feb 23, 2001

Bear, Judy. Stages of Grief. Cancer Survivors.org.: 3/30/2005

Bingham R. And Death Shall Set Ye Free. Neonatal Network. 15(2): 81-82; 1996

Brant J.M. The Art of Palliative care: Living with Hope, Dying with Dignity. Oncology Nursinf Forum 25(6): 995-1004; 1998

Byock, I. Dying Well: Peace and Possibilities at the End of Life. Riverhead Trade; 1998.

Callanan M. Farewell Messages. AJN. 94(5) 19-20; 1994

Callanan M. Breaking the Silence. 94(1): 22-23; 1994

Clingerman E. M. Bereavement Tasks for Nursing Students. Nurse Educator. 21(3): 19-22; 1996

Coberly M. Sacred Passage: How to Provide Fearless, Compassionate Care for the Dying. Shambhala. Boston; 2002

Coolican MB, Stark J, Doka KJ, Corr CA, Education About Death, Dying and Bereavement in Nursing Programs. Nurse Educator 19(6) 35-40; 1994

Costello J. Helping Relatives Cope with the Grieving Process. Professional Nurse 11(2): 89-92; 1995

Counsel C, Guin P Exploring Family Needs During Withdrawl of Life Support in Critically Ill Patients. Critical Care Nursing Clinics of North America. 14(2): 187-191; 2002

Hospice of Mid-Coast Maine. A Call to Action. www.curtis library. com

Czerwiec M. When a Loved One is Dying Families Talk About Nursing Care. AJN. 96(5): 32-36; 1996

Deffner JM, Bell SK, Nurses' Death Anxiety, Comfort Level During Communication with patients and families Regarding Death and Exposure to Communication Education. Journal For Nurses in Staff Development. 21(1): 19-23; 2005

Degner LF, Gow CM. Evaluations of Death Education in Nursing. Cancer Nursing. 11(3): 151-159; 1988

Degner LF, Gow CM. Preparing Nurses for Care of the Dying. Cancer Nursing. 11(3): 160-169; 1988

Despelder LA, Strickland AL. The Last dance: Encountering Death and Dying. 2nd Edition. Mayfield Publishing Co. Mountainview; 1999

Dombeck MB. Dream Telling: A Means of Spiritual Awareness. Holistic Nursing Practice; 1995

Downy V, Bengiamin M, HeuerL, Juhl N. Dying Babies and Associated Stress in NICU Nurses. Neonatal Network. 14(1): 41-45; 1995

Dunaway P. Decisions to Discontinue Intensive Therapy, Influencing Factors and Approaches to Decision Making. Intensive Care Nursing. 4: 106-111; 1988

Dyer ID. Breaking the News: Informing Visitors that a Patient has Died. Intensive and Critical care Nursing. 9: 2-10; 1993

Field D. Nurses Accounts of the Terminally Ill on a Coronary Care Unit. Intensive Care Nursing. 5: 114-122; 1989

Franklin P. Critical Moments: Death Challenges a Healer. AJN 92(5): 16B-16D; 1992

Gaglione KM. Assessing and Intervening with Families of CCU Patients. Nursing Clinics of North America 19(3): 427-433; 1984

Greifzus S. Grieving Families Need Your Help. RN September 22-28; 1996

Grafton HA. The Trauma Nurses Role with Families in Crisis. Critical Care Nurse April: 35-43; 1994

Hurtig WA, Stewin L. The Effect of Death Education and Experience in Nursing Students' Attitude Towards Death. Journal of Advanced Nursing. 15: 29-34; 1990

Jezierski MB. We Hurt Too. Nursing April: 160; 1988

Joel LA. Deferring to the Dying. AJN 94(2): 7; 1994

Johnson L. Communication: The Key to Crisis Prevention in Pediatric Death. Critical Care Nurse Dec: 23-27; 1992

Jones I, Kirby A, Ormiston P, Yogesh L, Kung-Kim C, Rout J, Nagel J, WardmanL, Hamilton S. The Needs of the Patient Dying of Chronic Obstructive Lung Disease. Family Practice. 21(3): 310-313; 2004

Kasman DL. When a Heart Stops. Annals of Internal Medicine. 120(5): 432-433; 1994.

Kesler D. The Needs of the Dying. Geriatric Times. May/June Vol 11, no. 3; 2001

Kirchhoff KT. Promoting a Peaceful Death in The ICU. Critical Care Nursing Clinics of North America. 14(2): 201-206; 2002

Kirkwood NA. A Hospital Handbook on Multi-culturalism and Religion. Australia: Millenium Books; 1993

Langford JM. Death and Dying in Ethnic America: Findings in Lao Lum, Khma, Hmong, Kher, and CHam Communities. The Cross Care Cultural Program. Seattle; 2000

Leash RM. Death Notification: Practical Guidelines for Health Care Professionals. Critical Care Nurse. 19(1): 21-34; 1996

Lewis CS. A Grief Observed. Harper. San Francisco; 2001

Lightfoot S. What do I Say? Emergency December 22-23; 1991.

Lipson JG, Dribble SL, Minarik PA. Culture and Nursing Care: a Pocket Guide. The Regents, University of California. San Francisco; 1996

London F. How We Coped With a Colleague's Death. RN. December 14-15; 1988

Mantell S. www.relaxintuit.com

Martinson IM. Funeral Rituals in Taiwan and Korea. Oncology Nursing Forum. 25(10):1756-60; 1998

Marttochhio BC. Grief and Bereavement: Healing Through Hurt. Nursing Clinics of North America. 20(2): 327-341; 1985

Mazanec P, Tyler MK. Cultural Considerations in End-of-Life Care. AJN 103(3): 50-58; 2003

McClement SE, Degner LF. Expert Nursing Behaviors in the Care of the Dying Adult in the Intensive Care Unit. Heart & Lung. 24(5): 408-419; 1995

McCorkle R. Death Education. Cancer Nursing. 11(3): 150; 1988

McKerracher B. How to Lend Support in a Crisis. Nursing November" 62-64; 1990

McKerron LC. Dealing with the Stress of Caring for the Dying in Intensive Care Units: An Overview. Intensive Care Nursing. 7:219-222; 1991

McLaughlan CAJ. Handling Distressed Realtives and Breaking Bad News. BMJ. 301: 149-150, 1145-1149; 1990

Meinyer EK. Grief, Communication and Culture at the End of Life. End of Life Nursing Education Consortium. www.netce. com; 2002

Mings D. Developing a Nursing Caregiver Bereavement Resource Package. The 1995 Schering lecture. 121-129; 1995

Mount BM Dealing with Our Losses. Journal of Clinical Oncology. 4(7): 1127-1134; 1986

Neuhaus RJ. As I Lay Dying. Basic Books. New York; 2002

Nishimoto P. Venturing into the Unknown: Cultural Beliefs About Death & Dying. Oncology Nursing Forum. 23(6): 889-894; 1996

Pitorak EF. Care at the Time of Death. AJN. 103(7) 42-52; 2003

Post-White J, Ceronsky C, Kreitzer MJ, Nickelson K, Drew D, Mackey KW, Koopmeiners L, GutKnecht S. Hope, Spirituality, Sense of Coherence, and Quality of Life in Patients with Cancer. Oncology Nursinf Forum. 23(10): 1571-1579; 1996

Rando TA. <u>Grief, Dying and Death: Clinical Interventions for Caregivers.</u> Research Press Co. Champaign; 1984

Rushton CH, SabatierK, Gaunines J. <u>Uniting to Improve End-of-Life Care.</u> Nursing Management 34(1): 30-33; 1984

Sammarino D. <u>Section 6: Dealing with the Dying Patient, Supportive Care and the Quality of Life of the Cancer Patient</u>. JB LIppincott, Philadelphia; 1993

Sherman DW. In M.L. Matzo and D.W. Sherman <u>Palliative Care Nursing: Quality Care to End of Life.</u> Springer Publishing Co. New York; 2001

Solomon NRZ. <u>Death and Dying in Ethnic America: Findings in Eritrean, Oromo, and Somali Communities.</u> The Cross Cultural Health Care Program. Seattle; 2000

Spitzer WJ, Burke L. A Critical-Incident Stress Debriefing Program for Hospital-Based Health Care Personnel. Health and Social Work. 18(2) 149-156; 1993

Stewart BP. <u>My Patient Died Today</u>. AJN 94(6): 80; 1994

Taylor PB. <u>Fostering Farewell</u>. Nursing. January: 54-57; 1996

Thompson DG. <u>Support for the Grieving Family: A Case Study</u>. Neonatal Network. 11(6): 73-75; 1992

Ufema J. <u>At a Loss for Words</u>. Nursing. January: 22; 1996

Ufema J. <u>What Color is Death?</u> Nursing. February: 28-29; 1996

Ufema J. <u>Tricks of the Trade.</u> Nursing March: 20; 1996

Van Bloch L. <u>Breaking the Bad News When Sudden Death Occurs</u>. Social Work in Health care. 23(4): 91-97; 1996

Villarruel AM, Ortiz de Montello B. Culture and Pain: A Mesoamerican Perspective. Advances in Nursing Science. 15(1): 21-32; 1992

Virani R, Sofer D. Improving the Quality of End-of-Life Care. AJN, 103(5) 52-60; 2003

Walker RJ, Pkmeroy EC, McNeil JS, Franklin C. Anticipatory Grief in AIDs: Strategies for Intervening with Caregivers. Health and Social Work. 21(1): 49-57; 1996

Youll JW. The Bridge Beyond: Strengthening Nursing Practice in Attitudes Towards Death, Dying, and the Terminally Ill, and Helping Spopuses of Critically Ill Patients. Internsive Care Nursing 5: 88-94; 1989

Zerwekh J. The Truth-Tellers: How Hospice Nurses Help Patients Confront Death. AJN. 94(2) 3`-34; 1994

Zunin LM, Zunin HS. The Art of Condolence. Harper Perennia. New York; 1992

Recommended Reading, References on Saints, quotes of Saints and Heaven.

The Bible, Douay-Rheims version. Baronius Press, London; 2007.

The Amplified Bible. Zondervan, Grand Rapids; 1987.

The New Catholic Answer Bible, NAB. Our Sunday Visitor Publication, Huntington; 1997.

The Four Volume Liturgy of the Hours. Catholic Book Publishing Co., New York; 1975.

Julian of Norwich. Showings. Paulist Press. Bronx; 1978.

Thomas a Kempis, translated by Clare L. Fitzpatrick. <u>The Imitation of Christ</u>. Catholic Book Publishing Co., New York; 1993.

Knotts, Betty I. <u>The Imitation of Christ by Thomas a Kempis</u>. William Collins and Sons (Font Books) Great Britain; 1984.—(Excellent for reading with books on Therese)

Michael Freze SFO. <u>They Bore The Wounds of Christ</u>. Our Sunday Visitor Publications, Huntington; 1989.

Rene Laurentin, translated by John Lynch, SM and Ronald DesRosiers, SM. <u>Bernadette in Her Own Words.</u> Pauline Books and Media, Boston; 2000.

St. Gertrude and a religious of her monastery. Translated by the Poor Clares of Kenmare. <u>The Life and Revelations of St. Gertrude The Great.</u> Tan Books and Publishers, Rockford; 2002.

Sr. Josepha Menendez. <u>The Way of Divine Love.</u> Tan Books and Publishers, Rockford; 2002.

<u>Diary of Saint Maria Faustina Kowalska.</u> Marian Press, Stockbridge; 1981.

Abbe Theodore Ratisbonne. <u>St. Bernard of Clairvaux</u>. Tan Books (Sadlier) Rockford; 1855.

Translated by Colledge, Edmund O.S.A. Walsh, James, S.J. <u>Julian of Norwich—Showings</u>. Paulist, Mahwah; 1978.

St. Therese, translated by John Clarke, OCD. <u>Story of a Soul.</u> ICS Publications, Washington; 1996.

C. Bernard Ruffin. <u>Padre Pio: The True Story</u>. Our Sunday Visitor Publishing, Huntington; 1991.

Gianluigi Pasquale. <u>Secrets of a Soul-Padre Pio's Letters to His Spiritual Directors</u>. Pauline Books, Boston; 2003

By Father John Croiset, SJ, translated by Father Patrick O'Connell, BD. <u>Devotion to The Sacred Heart of Jesus.</u> Tan Books and Publishers, Rockford; 1988.

Farber, Fredrick, William, D.D. <u>The Precious Blood.</u> Tan Publishing, Rockford; 1959.

Translated by Marison Fiscar. <u>Venerable Mary of Agreda-The City of God.</u> Tan Publishing, Rockford; 1978.

Translated by Raphael Brown, Benen Fahy, Placid Hermann, Paul Oligny, Nesta de Robeck, Leo Sherley-Price. <u>St. Francis of Assisi Omnibus of Sources</u>. Franciscan Press, Quincy; 1991.

Regis J. Armstrong OFM cap<u>. The Lady. Clare of Assisi, Early Documents.</u> New City Press. New York; 2006.

Blessed Raymond of Capua, translated by George Lamb. <u>The Life of St. Catherine of Siena.</u> Tan Books and Publishers, Rockford; 2003.

Catherine of Siena, <u>The Dialogue. (one of "The Classics of Western Spirituality")</u> translated by Suzanne Noffke, OP. Paulist Press Inc., 1978; Mahwah; 1980.

Jean-Jacques Antier, translated by Claire Quintal. <u>Teresa of Avila, God Alone Suffices</u>. Pauline Books and Media, Boston; 1993.

Francisco de Osuna. <u>The Third Spiritual Alphabet</u>, translated by Mary E. Giles. Paulist Press, New York; 1981

<u>The 33 Doctors of the Church.</u> Fr. Christopher Rengers, OFM. Tan Publishing, Rockford; 2000.

St. Teresa of Avila, translated by Kieran Kavanaugh, OCD and Otilio Rodroquez, OCD. <u>Writings of St. Teresa of Avila</u>, in Three Volumes. ICS Publications, Washington; 1985.

Margaret Rowe. <u>God is Love. Saint Theresa Margaret: Her Life.</u> ICS Pub, Washington; 2003.

Peggy Wilkinson OCDS. <u>Finding the Mystic Within You.</u> ICS Publications, Washington; 1999.

<u>Fire Within</u>, by Father Thomas Dubay. Ignatius Press, San Francisco; 1989.

St. John of the Cross, translated by E. Allison Peers.

St. John of the Cross. <u>Dark Night of the Soul.</u> Image Books/ Doubleday, New York; 2005

Translated by Kavanaugh, Kieran, OCD. Rodriguez, Otilio OCD. <u>The Complete Works of St. John of the Cross.</u> ICS Publications, Washington;1991.

Translated by Mother M. Philip IBVM. <u>The Spiritual Direction of St. Claude De La Columbiere</u>. Ignatius Press, San Francisco; 1998.

Rt. Rev. Dom Vitalis, Lehodey OCR. <u>The Ways of Mental Prayer.</u> (orig. 1924) Tan Publishing, Rockford; 1982.

P. Marie-Eugene OCD. <u>I Want to See God.</u> Christian Classics, Allen; 1958.

P. Marie-Eugene OCD. <u>I am a Daughter of the Church.</u> Christian Classics, Allen; 1997.

Sullivan, Kathryn, R.S.G. Paul-Marie of the Cross. <u>Carmelite Spirituality in the Teresian Tradition.</u>

ICS Publications, Washington;1997.

Sr. Mary of St. Peter, edited by Dorothy Scallan, translated by Fr, Emeric Scallan, STB. The Golden Arrow. Tan Publishing, Rockford; 1954.

Harvey Egan, SJ. What are They Saying About Mysticism. (a Catholic view from, "Mysticism" by Evelyn Underhill. Bracken Books, London; 1942) Paulist Press, New York; 1982.

Father Gabriel of Mary Magdalene OCD. Divine Intimacy, TAN Books & Publishers, Rockford; 1964.

Rev. Placido Fabrini. The Life and Works of St. Mary Magdalen De-Pazzi. translated by Rev Antonio Isoleri, Philadelphia; 1900.

Catechism of the Catholic Church Image Book/Doubleday, New York; 1995.

The Mirror of Perfection by St. Bonaventure translated Robert Steele, EP Dutton Co., New York;1951

The Soul's Journey into God, The Tree of Life, The Life of St. Francis by Bonaventure translated by Ewert Cousins. Paulist Press Inc., Mahwah; 1978.

Phillip Keller. The Classic Works of Phillip Keller A Shepherd Looks at the 23 Psalm, A Shepherd Looks at The Good Shepherd and His Sheep. Family Christian Press. Grand Rapids, 1970-78.

Purgatorian Manual. Catholic Men for Christ the King. PO Box 7001 Wantagh, NY 11793-0601

Susan Tassone. Thirty-Day Devotions for the Holy Souls. Our Sunday Visitor Publications.

Purgatory. Father Frederick William Faber. TAN Publishing.

Fr. John A. Hardon, S.J. Devotion to the Poor Souls.

Rev, Nageleisen. <u>Charity for The Suffering Souls,</u> Rockford. Tan Books and Publishers; 1977

J Moorman & M Habig. <u>St. Francis of Assisi, Omnibus of Sources</u>. Franciscan Press, Quincy; 1972.

Giuliana Cavallini. <u>St. Martin de Porres, Apostle of Charity</u>. TAN Books & Publishers, Rockford; 1963

Rev. Placido Fabrini. <u>The Life and Works of St. Mary Magdalen De-Pazzi</u>. Rev. Antonio Isoleri Miss. Ap. Philadelphia; 1900.

Father Conrad De Meester, ODC. <u>Elizabeth of the Trinity, The Complete Works Vol I & II.</u> ICS Publications, Washington; 1995.

Recommended Reading on St. Therese of Lisieux, and Audio and Visual Material Books:

Translated by S.L. Emery, <u>Poems of Sr. Therese, Carmelite of Lisieux, known as the "Little Flower of Jesus".</u> Note: This was published before her canonization! This is available online as a free download via catholicfirst.com or ccel.org.

Fulton Sheen. <u>Archbishop Fulton Sheen's St. Therese.</u> Irving. Basilica Press; 2007.

Franciscan Friars of the Immaculate. <u>St. Therese: Doctor of the Little Way.</u> Waite Park. Park Press Inc.; 1997.

Father Jean C. J. d'Elbee. <u>I Believe in Love</u>. Chicago. Franciscan herald Press; 2001.

Guy Gaucher, Auxilary Bishop of Bayeux and Lisieux. <u>John and Therese: Flames of Love.</u> New York. St. Paul's Press; 1999.

Frederick L Miller STD. <u>The Trial of Faith of St. Therese of Lisieux.</u> New York. Alaba House; 1998.

Guy Gaucher, Auxilary Bishop of Bayeux and Lisieux. <u>The Passion of Therese of Lisieux</u>. New York Crossroad; 2006.

John Udris. <u>Holy Daring.</u> Boston. Pauline Books; 2007.

Conrad De Meester. <u>With Empty Hands.</u> New York. Burns and Oates; 2002.

Conrad De Meester. <u>The Power of Confidence</u>. New York. Alba House; 1969.

Patrick Ahern, Bishop. <u>Maurice and Therese.</u> New York. Doubleday Books; 1998.

St. Therese, translated by John Clarke OCD. <u>Story of a Soul</u>. Washington. ICS Publications; 1996.

St. Therese, translated by John Clarke OCD. <u>Letters of St. Therese of Lisieux, Volume I.</u> Washington. ICS Publications; 1972.

St. Therese, translated by John Clarke OCD. <u>Letters of St. Therese of Lisieux, Volume II.</u> Washington. ICS Publications; 1974.

St. Therese, translated by John Clarke OCD. <u>St. Therese of Lisieux, Her Last Conversations.</u> Washington. ICS Publications; 1977.

Father Vernon Johnson. <u>Spiritual Childhood, The Spirituality of St. Therese of Lisieux.</u> San Francisco. Ignatius; 2001.

St. Therese, translated by Susan Conroy and David J. Dwyer. <u>The Plays of St. Therese of Lisieux</u>. Washington. ICS Publications;2008.

St. Therese, translated by Aletheia Kane OCD. <u>The Prayers of St. Therese of Lisieux.</u> Washington. ICS Publications;1997.

Christopher O'Mahony. <u>St. Therese of Lisieux by Those who Knew Her</u>. Dublin. Veritas Publications, 1975.

Sr. Genevieve of The Holy Face (Celine Martin) <u>My Sister Saint Therese</u>. Rockford. Tan Books and Publishers; 1997.

Ida Friederike Gorres. <u>The Hidden Face: A Study of</u> St. Therese of Lisieux. San Francisco. Ignatius; 2003.

Joseph F. Schmidt. <u>Everything is Grace: The Life and Way of Therese of Lisieux</u>. Ijamsville. The Word Among Us Press; 2007.

L'Abbe Andre Combs. The Spirituality of St. Therese. New York. P.J. Ken edy and Sons; 1950.

L'Abbe Andre Combs. St. Therese and Suffering: The Spirituality of St. Therese in its Essence. New York. P.J. Kennedy and Sons; 1951.

John Sullivan OCD. Experiencing St. Therese Today. Washington. ICS Publications;1990.

Bernard bro, OP. The Spirituality of St. Therese of Lisieux. Westminister. Christian Classics; 1980.

Ann Laforest, OCD. The Way to Love, Therese of Lisieux. Franklin. Sheed & Ward; 2000.

Arthur Cavanaugh. Therese, The Saint Who Loved Us. New York. Paulist Press; 2003.

Dorothy Scallan. The Whole World Will Love Me. The Life of St. Therese of the Child Jesus and the Holy Face. Rockford. Tan Books and Publishers;2005.

Thomas R. Nevin. Therese of Lisieux, God's Gentle Warrior. New York. Oxford University Press; 2006.

Elizabeth Ficocelli. Shower of Heavenly Roses. Stories of the Intercession of St. Therese of Lisieux.
New York. Crossroad Publishing Co.; 2004.

Bishop A. A. Noser, SVD, DD. Joy in Suffering. Rockford. Tan Books and Publishers; 2006.

Marie-Eugene of the Child Jesus. Under the Torrent of His Love. Staten Island. Alba House; 2004.

Jean Guitton. The Spiritual Genius of Saint Therese of Lisieux. Liguori. Ligouri/Triumph; 1997.

Susan Leslie. <u>The Happiness of God.</u> Staten Island. St Pauls/Alba; 1988

M. Pascale Ducrocq. <u>Therese of Lisieux: Vocation of Love.</u> Staten Island. St Pauls/Alba; 1982.

Pierre Descouvement. <u>Therese of Lisieux and Marie of the Trinity.</u> Staten Island. St Pauls/Alba. House; 1997.

Francois Jamart OCD. <u>Complete Spiritual Doctrine of St. Therese of Lisieux</u>. Staten Island. St Pauls/Alba House; 1977.

Fr. Charles P. Connor. <u>The Saint for the Third Millenium St. Therese of Lisieux.</u> Staten Island. St Pauls/Alba. House; 2007.

Steven Payne OCD. <u>Saint Therese of Lisieux Doctor of the Universal Church</u>. Staten Island. St Pauls/Alba. House; 2002.

Patricia O'Connor. <u>The Inner Life of St. Therese of Lisieux</u>. Orlando. Our Sunday Visitor; 1997.

Pere Marie-Eugene of the Child Jesus, OCD. <u>Where the Spirit Breathes.</u> Staten Island. St Pauls/Alba. House; 1998.

Dodds, Monica. <u>Praying in The Presence of Our Lord with Therese of Lisieux.</u> Sunday Visitor Publishing, Huntington; 2004. (Good for contemplation)

Cliff Ermatinger. <u>St. Therese of Lisieux: Spouse and Victim.</u> ICS. Washington; 2010

<u>Note: The following are nice little books of quotes of Therese.</u>

Translated by an Irish Carmelite. <u>Thoughts of St. Therese</u>. Rockford. Tan Books and Publishers; 1988.

John P.McClernon. <u>Sermon in a Sentence Series: St. Therese of Lisieux.</u> San Francisco. Ignatius; 2002.

Francis Broome, CSP. <u>The Little Way for Every Day.</u> New York. Paulist Press; 2006.

Judith A.Bauer. <u>Therese of Lisieux In My Own Words.</u> Liguori, Liguori Books; 2005.

John Nelson. <u>The Little Way of</u> St. Therese of Lisieux. Liguori, Liguori Books; 1998.

Cynthia Cavnar. <u>Spiritual Treasures From St. Therese of Lisieux</u>. Ijamsville. The Word Among Us Press; 2007.

Marc Foley, OCD. <u>The Path of Merciful Love. 99 Sayings by Therese of Lisieux</u>. Hyde Park. New City Press; 2006.

James McCaffrey, OCD. <u>Fire of Love, Praying with Therese of Lisieux</u>. Boston. Pauline Press; 2004.

Father Charles Arminjon. <u>The End of the Present World and the Mysteries of the Future Life.</u> Manchester. Sophia Institue Press; 2008.

-Cassettes:

<u>This Child.</u> ICS Publications.

-CDs:

John P.McClernon. <u>Praying the Rosary with</u> St. Therese of Lisieux. Oklahoma City. Summa Enterprises; 2005.

John Welsh, O.Carm. <u>Therese: The Discovery of Merciful Love</u>, CD # 152, CC Communications (see ICS)

Dr, Mary Frohich. <u>Therese and the Priesthood.</u> CD# 144 CC Communications (see ICS)

Kieran Kavanaugh, OCD. <u>The Little Way</u>. CD# 133 CC Communications (see ICS)

Kieran Kavanaugh, OCD. <u>The Revolution of Therese</u>. CD# 130 CC Communications (see ICS)

John Sullivan, OCD. <u>Empathy: The Key to Therese's Little Way</u>. CD# 115 CC Communications (see ICS)

Keith J. Egan, T.O. Carm. <u>Therese: Doctor of The Church</u>. CD# 137 CC Communications (see ICS)

John Welsh, O.Carm. <u>The Discovery of merciful Love</u>. CD # 140 CC Communications (see ICS)

Steven Payne, OCD. <u>Reflections on the Doctorate of St. Therese.</u> CD # 154 AQ CC Communications (see ICS)

Daniel Chowning, OCD. <u>Dark Fire: The Prayer of St. Therese.</u> CD# 165 CC Communications (see ICS)

-DVDs:

<u>Miracle of St. Therese.</u> San Francisco. Ignatius; 1959.

Leonardo Defillipis. <u>Therese: Ordinary Girl, Extraordinary Soul</u>. Xenon Pictures. Luke Films Inc. 2004-2006.

The sacrifice I love, the cross is my desire
O! deign (stoop down) to summon me, full ready now am I
O Master, for Thy love to suffer I aspire
Jesus, my well-Beloved, for Thee I long to die.

If bitter pain you life invade,
Threatening gladness to destroy
Of anguish may delight be made.
Suffer for God! Tis purest joy.

By the Cross sinners find relief.

To live by love is not on earth to rest.
E'en though on Thabor might our dwelling be;
But tis to climb to Calvary's rugged crest,
Holding the Cross . . . our hearts sole treasury.
In realms celestial, joy hath endless sway
There trial shall no more the spirit prove;
But here below, in anguish deep I pray
To live by love.

St. Therese & Suffering, Abbe Andre Combes, NY, PJ Kennedy & Sons; 1952
(from St. Therese's Poems). S.L. Emery excellent translator of her first book
of poems, published before her canonization.

Addendum—Words from Paul.

Cor. II: 4:7-5:8

This treasure we possess in earthen vessels to make it clear that its surpassing power comes from God and not from us. We are afflicted in every way possible, but we are not crushed; full of doubts, we never despair. We are persecuted but never abandoned; we are struck down but never destroyed. Continually we carry about in our bodies the dying of Jesus, so that in our bodies the life of Jesus may also be revealed.

While we live we are constantly being delivered to death for Jesus' sake, so that the life of Jesus may be revealed in our mortal flesh. Death is at work in us, but life in you. We have the spirit of faith of which the scripture says, "Because I believed, I spoke out."

We believe and so we speak, knowing that He who raised up the Lord Jesus will raise us up along with Jesus and place both us and you in His presence.

Indeed everything is ordered to your benefit, so that the grace bestowed in abundance may bring greater glory to God because they who give thanks are many.

We do not lose heart, because our inner being is renewed each day even though our body is being destroyed at the same time. The present burden of our trial is light enough, and earns for us an eternal weight of glory beyond all comparison. We do not fix our gaze on what is seen but on what is unseen. What is seen is transitory, what is unseen lasts for ever.

Indeed we know that when the earthly tent in which we dwell is destroyed we have a dwelling provided for us by God, a dwelling in the heavens, not made by hands but to last forever. We groan while we are here, even as we yearn to have our heavenly habitation envelop us. This it will, provided we are found clothed and not naked. While we live in our present tent we groan; we are weighed down because we do not wish to be stripped naked but rather to have the heavenly dwelling envelop us, so that what is mortal may be absorbed by life. God has fashioned us for this very thing and has given us the Spirit as a pledge of it.

Therefore we continue to be confident. We know that while we dwell in the body we are away from the Lord. We walk by faith, not by sight. I repeat, we are full of confidence and would much rather be away from the body and at home with the Lord.

Philippians 3:7-4:1, 4-9

Those things I used to count as gain I have now reappraised as loss in the light of Christ. I have come to rate all as loss in the light of the surpassing knowledge of my Lord, Jesus Christ. For His sake I have forfeited everything; I have counted all else rubbish so that Christ may be my wealth and I may be in Him, not having any justice of my own based on observance of the law. The justice I possess is that which comes from faith in Christ. It has its origin in God and is based on faith. I wish to know Christ and the power flowing from His resurrection; likewise to know how to share in His sufferings by being formed into the pattern of His death. Thus do I hope that I might arrive at resurrection from the dead.

It is not that I have reached it yet, or have already finished my course; but I am racing to grasp the prize if possible, since I have been grasped by Christ. Brothers, I do not think of myself as having reached the finish line. I give no thought to what lies behind but push on to what is ahead. My entire attention is on the finish line as I run towards the prize to which God calls me—life on high in Christ Jesus.

St. Bonaventure of Potenza on the Life of Perfection

The law of the Lord teaches us what we are to do, what we are to avoid, what we should pray for, what we should desire, what we should fear. It teaches us to be without sin and without reproach. It teaches us to keep our promises and to weep over our sins. It teaches us to despise the things of the world and to reject things of the flesh. Finally, it teaches us how to turn our whole heart, our whole mind to Jesus Christ alone.

Compared to this teaching all the wisdom of this world is foolish and empty. He who is no forgetful listener but one who carries out the law diligently is truly wise, truly happy. But to eradicate vice, to make progress in grace, to achieve the highest perfection of virtue we can name nothing better, think of nothing more useful than love.

Such is the power of love that it alone opens heaven, gives us hope, and makes us loved by God . . .

Examine carefully the kind of love your Beloved seeks from you. He wants you to give your whole heart, your whole soul, your whole mind to His love in such a way, that in your whole heart, your whole soul in your whole mind absolutely no one has any part together with Him.

I most strongly recommend reading St. Therese of Lisieux.

Though on first reading she seems to many too sweet, she is a warrior

and if one persists, she will remain with you and escort you through

the dark night, into the eternal day.

Editor, Bro Patrick Bernard Francis Gillen unworthy SFO

Act of Oblation to Merciful Love, by
Saint Therese of Lisieux

Offering of myself as a Victim of Holocaust to God's Merciful Love

O My God! Most Blessed Trinity, I desire to Love You and make you Loved, to work for the glory of Holy Church by saving souls on earth and liberating those suffering in purgatory. I desire to accomplish Your will perfectly and to reach the degree of glory You have prepared for me in Your Kingdom. I desire, in a word, to be saint, but I feel my helplessness and I beg You, O my God! to be Yourself my Sanctity!
Since You loved me so much as to give me Your only Son as my Savior and my Spouse, the infinite treasures of His merits are mine. I offer them to You with gladness, begging You to look upon me only in the Face of Jesus and in His heart burning with Love.
I offer You, too, all the merits of the saints (in heaven and on earth), their acts of Love, and those of the holy angels. Finally, I offer You, O Blessed Trinity! the Love and merits of the Blessed Virgin, my Dear Mother. It is to her I abandon my offering, begging her to present it to You. Her Divine Son, my Beloved Spouse, told us in the days of His mortal life: "Whatsoever you ask the Father in my name He will give it to you!" I am certain, then, that You will grant my desires; I know, O my God! that the more You want to give, the more You make us desire. I feel in my heart immense desires and it is with confidence I ask You to come and take possession of my soul. Ah! I cannot receive Holy Communion as often as I desire, but, Lord, are You not all-powerful? Remain in me as in a tabernacle and never separate Yourself from Your little victim.
I want to console You for the ingratitude of the wicked, and I beg of you to take away my freedom to displease You. If through weakness I sometimes fall, may Your Divine Glance cleanse my soul immediately, consuming all my

imperfections like the fire that transforms everything into itself.

I thank You, O my God! for all the graces You have granted me, especially the grace of making me pass through the crucible of suffering. It is with joy I shall contemplate You on the Last Day carrying the sceptre of Your Cross. Since You deigned to give me a share in this very precious Cross, I hope in heaven to resemble You and to see shining in my glorified body the sacred stigmata of Your Passion.

After earth's Exile, I hope to go and enjoy You in the Fatherland, but I do not want to lay up merits for heaven. I want to work for Your Love Alone with the one purpose of pleasing You, consoling Your Sacred Heart, and saving souls who will love You eternally.

In the evening of this life, I shall appear before You with empty hands, for I do not ask You, Lord, to count my works. All our justice is stained in Your eyes. I wish, then, to be clothed in Your own Justice and to receive from Your Love the eternal possession of Yourself. I want no other Throne, no other Crown but You, my Beloved!

Time is nothing in Your eyes, and a single day is like a thousand years. You can, then, in one instant prepare me to appear before You.

In order to live in one single act of perfect Love, <u>I OFFER MYSELF AS A VICTIM OF HOLOCAUST TO YOUR MERCIFUL LOVE</u>, Asking You to consume me incessantly, allowing the waves of infinite tenderness shut up within You to overflow into my soul, and that thus I may become a martyr of Your Love, O my God!

May this martyrdom, after having prepared me to appear before You, finally cause me to die and may my soul take its flight without any delay into the eternal embrace of Your Merciful Love.

I want, O my Beloved, at each beat of my heart to renew this offering to You an infinite number of times, until the shadows having disappeared I may be able to tell You of my Love in an Eternal Face to Face!

Marie, Françoise, Thérèse of the Child Jesus and the Holy Face, unworthy Carmelite religious.
This 9th day of June, Feast of the Most Holy Trinity, In the year of grace, 1895 *from Story of A Soul,*

From a sermon by St. Bernard, abbot

. . . Come, let us at length spur ourselves on. We must rise again with Christ, we must seek the world which is above and set our minds on the things of heaven. Let us long for those who are longing for us, hasten to those who are waiting for us, and ask those who look for our coming to intercede for us. (As we pray for one another here below, it is all right to ask the Saints intercession). We should not only want to be with the saints, we should also hope to possess their happiness. While we desire to be in their company, we must also earnestly seek to share in their glory. Do not imagine that there is anything harmful in such an ambition as this; there is no danger in setting our hearts on such glory.

When we commemorate the saints we are inflamed with another yearning: that Christ our life may also appear to us as He appeared to them and that we may one day share in His glory. Until then we see Him, not as He is, but as He became for our sake. He is our head, crowned, not with glory, but with the thorns of our sins . . . When Christ comes again, His death shall no longer be proclaimed, and we shall know that we also have died, and that our life is hidden with Him. The glorious head of the Church will appear and His glorified members will shine in splendor with Him, when He forms this lowly body anew into such glory as belongs to Himself, its head.

Therefore, we should aim at attaining this glory with a wholehearted and prudent desire. That we might rightly hope and strive for such blessedness, we must seek the prayers of the saints . . .

St John of the Cross—The Spiritual Canticle, stanza 11

Since the Israelites were not so fortified in love or so close to God through love, they feared to die on seeing Him. But because now in the law of grace the soul can see god when separated from the body, the desire to live but a short while and die in order to see Him is more perfect. And even if this were false, the soul loving God as intensely as this one does would not fear to die from seeing Him. True love receives all things that come from the Beloved-prosperity, adversity, even chastisement-with the same evenness of soul, since they are His will. And they afford her joy and delight because, as St. John says: "perfect charity casts out all fear." (1 Jn 4:18).

Death cannot be bitter to the soul that loves, for in it she finds all the sweetness and delight of love. The thought of death cannot sadden her, for what she finds is that gladness accompanies this thought. Neither can the thought of death be burdensome and painful to her, for death will put an end to all her sorrows and afflictions and be the beginning of all her bliss. She thinks of death as her friend and bridegroom, and at the thought of it she rejoices as if she would over the thought of her betrothal and marriage, and she longs for the day and the hour of her death more than earthly kings long for kingdoms and principalities.

This is all so very true and reflected in the thoughts of Bernadette, Therese of Lisieux, Teresa of Avila, Catherine of Siena, Francis of Assisi, Bonaventure, and so many other Saints and mystics. Love is merely the door we go through to be with that one who loves us more than anyone else, more than we could have conceived of, forever.

Saint John of the Cross from a Spiritual Canticle-cited from the Breviary

. . . Would that men might come at last to see that it is quite impossible to reach the thicket of the riches and wisdom of God except by first entering the thicket of much suffering, in such a way that the soul finds there its consolation and desire. The soul that desires divine wisdom chooses first, and in truth, to enter the thicket of the cross.

Saint Paul therefore urges the Ephesians *not to grow weary in the midst of tribulations, but to be rooted and grounded in love, so that they may know with all the saints the breadth, the length, the height and the depth—to know what is beyond knowledge, the love of Christ, so as to be filled with the fullness of God.*

The gate that gives entry into these riches of His wisdom is the cross; because it is a narrow gate, while many seek the joys that can be gained through it, it is given to few to desire to pass through it.

I admit I used to dread suffering and pain, it stopped me from doing what I wanted. It robbed me of my sense of control. If I were honest I would admit it scared me as it posed a possible threat to life and control over my destiny. But I have learned one can choose to surrender all into God's hands. He is our loving Papa. We can just believe He will hold us in His arms and get us through it regardless of where it leads. As many people have found when we embrace His cross and suffering two things happen. 1) We are able to offer it up for the benefit of others. 2) We are able to share in His pain, (He choose to suffer for me), and so grow much closer to Him, much more aware of how very much I am loved. And Oh the Peace!—it passes all understanding.

What Comfort is There for Those Left Behind?

Throughout this book I have striven to show that suffering and dying are truly hidden blessings and graces. That when seen as acts which can be offered up for the redemption of others they can be better accepted and embraced with actual joy.

It is my hope that this will bring comfort to both the ill and their loved ones. I have added practical advice from over 25 years of lecturing on this subject to patients, family and health care providers.

But the other day I was reading a mystery novel. (It is amazing how God will use anything in life to talk with you.) And once again I saw the suffering of those who are left behind. Of the family and significant others who are left here, in this land of exile, while the patient, the one who died or is suffering, is separated from them by their disease, pain, lethargy, . . . departure.

I thought, "What about those, especially, those who <u>abruptly</u> lose loved ones? This may occur in an auto accident, a heart attack or stroke, . . . or more sadly perhaps through suicide or a violent crime."

In all these situations, even more so than with a more chronic scenario, the loved ones left behind are more . . . shattered, unprepared, by the experience. Even more do they ask . . . WHY? Why was this loved one taken away from me? Why did the tower of Siloam fall upon those eighteen, were they sinners, were their loved ones? (<u>Luke 13:2</u> And he answering said to them, *Think ye that these Galileans were sinners **beyond** all the Galileans because they suffered such things?*

<u>Luke 13:4</u> *Or those eighteen on whom the tower in Siloam fell and killed them, think ye that they were debtors **beyond** all the men who dwell in Jerusalem?)* The man born blind neither he nor his parents sinned.

Often we think or fear it happened because of something we did or they did, and so were punished. I remember a friend who had pancreatic cancer and a woman asked him, "Did you used to smoke?" and Doug said, "Yes, a long time ago." And she said, "Well, there you are, it's all your fault." I was shocked as a nurse practitioner and Christian to hear that anyone would say such a thing. But, people do, and often times in the still of the night we worry, was it my fault, was it their fault. We can become guilt ridden or depressed; or angry with them.

I believe it is never their fault or ours. I have known chain smokers who died of old age, and of non-smokers, who died of lung cancer.

Well, what about suicide? What about it, I tried suicide once, it was out of depression, believing way back then I would never be loved and the resulting pain was more than I could live with. After 40 years of reading and thinking hard about this I have come to a conclusion. People who commit suicide are not thinking right, if they did, they wouldn't commit suicide. And their whole reason is pain, a pain so bad that it causes them to forget about what this act will do to those left behind. It is not they don't care, it is that they are completely overwhelmed by pain, mental, emotional, physical.

What about murder, rape and murder? Was it because I let them go out, they strayed to a bad area. Something I did or did not do, something they did or did not do that resulted in it. Excuse me, No! It happened. No one planned for it to result in their death.

I remember a good friend and Emergency room nurse asking a doctor, "Why does God let these things happen?" The doctor looked at her with a kindly smile and said, "Oh Susie, think about it. God didn't want them to be hurt. He wanted them home with Him."

Would you pay $2500 dollars to go to Europe? Many, many do. I never could afford it. That's a lot to pay. Is pain and suffering and death a lot to pay? Yes! But OH! The rewards are wonderful beyond all comprehension.

What if, had they lived longer they would have done something bad that would have destroyed all their self esteem, their ability to love, to live a successful life . . . and God spared them this terrible hurt He knew was coming by calling them home. What if they had earned their reward. They were so good they earned their admittance to heaven.

He loves us so very much more than we do. More than we can ever understand. And this greatest of lovers is always right there with them. And I believe in the seconds they realize they are dying they reach out to Him and He takes their hand.

In the beginning I said that death could be an offering up that has such blessings attached. I lost a good friend who was like a son to me in 2002 in an auto accident. He was brain dead on arrival to the hospital. His parents carried out his wishes to have all his organs, eyes, kidneys, heart and lungs, donated to others. They were awed by what this young man of 20 accomplished, the lives he saved, the sight he restored, to so many others. More than many of us can hope to achieve in a life time. They have gone on with becoming very involved in promoting organ donation and have helped probably thousands of others, and found hope and joy for themselves. And, I have seen entire families reunited after years of issues, all brought to know the love of God and have more hope and strength; to go on through the rest of their lives and meet their own death with greater courage and hope, because of the experience of the death of a loved one and how it eventually ministered to their heart and soul.

Death is simply a door, like birth. A door to another, more wonderful, beautiful, bigger, and this time—eternal life. And doesn't that bring comfort? To KNOW that our loved ones are in a place more wonderful than we can ever imagine, happier than they have ever been, more loved than ever before; and that we can be with them there some day.

"But my husband, son, (whatever) was a bum, I know he must have gone to hell." I don't know that. I earned a white coat, never black robes. I am a nurse, and a minister, not a judge. Only Jesus judges. And He is so knowledgeable, and loving. None of us know what our loved one thought at the moment of death, I believe many, many repent of all wrong and desire His love. And, that the scriptures say is enough. And the last shall be first and the first last. And . . . I chose to pay those who only worked for me a second, as much as those who worked for me 100 years. Things like that God has said. So after 40 years I am very optimistic, especially since reading and getting to know Jesus, and Francis and Therese.

He wrote this because He loves you. I, His pencil, do too, and if I, such a small, insignificant, sinner, love you, how much infinitely more does an omnipotent, omnipresent, God who used me write it for you. You and all your loved ones are loved. Let us pray for each other, love each other, help each other, and be confident in His love for us.

In 2006-8 I gave the last of my lectures as a nurse practitioner and a nurse with 38 years experience with the suffering and dying and their loved ones. The Joint Commission of American Hospitals, JCAHO mandated lectures on death and dying as Americans felt the medical profession was letting them down in this area. I lectured to physicians, nurses and medical technicians and encouraged input from them.

I became totally disabled in May 2008 and each year finds me in greater suffering and closer to dying myself. In 2005 God gave me a need to read so very much of the lives of the Saints and the Catholic Church's Teachings. I had been reading the Bible for 39 years and the Breviary, Daily prayers that trace their origins to the Jewish traditions and Jesus, and were refined during the early religious orders and monasteries for 16. But now I felt lead, pushed, surrendered to reading all He guides me to. This continues to my wife's dismay at times. We are becoming engulfed in books. We call our bedroom the St. Peter Library Annex. I love the Gospels most, The Imitation of Christ by Thomas a Kempis and books on Therese, these I read daily; I especially also like the lives of the Saints i.e., Francis, Bernadette, Gertrude, Catherine of Siena, Mary Magdalen de Pazzi, Padre Pio, Teresa of Avila, John of the Cross, Faustina, Martin de Porres, Bernard and others all being good friends by now.

When I thought I finished this book God suggested I include the practical section as well. Finishing the Reference and Recommended Reading sections I thought I was through. Since then He keeps adding additional reflections that comfort me and so I hope will be of comfort to others. Know this He SO loves you! As Therese tells me repeatedly, "Everything is grace!" & "How can one fear such a tender friend as Jesus?"

From The Imitation of Christ by Thomas A Kempis- Translated by Betty I Knotts

Dear Lord and God! O Holy One, O Lover of my soul! When You come to my heart, all that is within me will leap up for joy. You are my glory, the rejoicing of my heart! You are my hope and refuge in my hour of peril.

Yet I am still weak in love, imperfect in goodness, and I need Your strength and comfort. So visit me often and teach me by Your holy discipline; free me from evil passions, and cure my heart of all its undisciplined emotions; then I shall be healthy and clean within, made fit for loving, strong for suffering, steadfast for enduring.

Love is a great thing, an altogether good gift, the only thing that makes burdens light and bears all that is hard with ease. It carries a weight without feeling it, and makes all that is bitter sweet and pleasant to the taste. The love of Jesus is noble and impels us to do great things; it continually stirs us up to desire the next stage in perfections. Love longs to be in the high places not held down by anything base. Love longs to be free, cut loose every earthly affection, so that the eyes of the soul may not be dimmed, so that no temporal advantage may entangle it and no obstacle cause it to fall.

Nothing is sweeter than love, nothing stronger, nothing higher, nothing broader; nothing is more lovely, nothing richer, nothing better in heaven or in earth. Love is born of God and it cannot rest anywhere but in God, beyond all created things. One who loves is born on wings; he runs, and is filled with joy; he is free and unrestricted. He gives all to receive all, and he has all in all; for beyond all things he rests in the highest thing, from whom streams all that is good. He does not consider the gift, but beyond all good things he turns himself to the giver. Love often knows no measure, but burns white-hot beyond all measure. Love knows no burden, counts up no toil; it aspires to do more than its strength allows; it does not plead impossibility, but considers it may do and can do all things. So it finds strength for anything; it completes and carries through great tasks where one who does not love would fail and fall. Love is vigilant, it sleeps without losing control; it is wearied without exhaustion, cramped without being crushed, alarmed without being destroyed. Like a living flame or a burning torch, it leaps up and passes safely through all. When a man loves he knows the meaning of that cry that sounds in the ears of God from the burning love of the soul: <u>My God, it cries, my Love! You are wholly mine, and I am wholly Yours!</u>

Expand my heart with love, so that the lips of my soul may taste how sweet it is to love, to melt in love and float upon a sea of love. Let me be gripped by love as I rise in adoration and wonder beyond the limits of my being! Let the song of love be on my lips as I follow my Love to the heights; let my soul, triumphant with love, faint in intensity of worship. May I love You more than myself, and myself only because of You; and in You let me love all those who truly love You. The law of love that shines from You gives us this command.

Love is eager, sincere, and kind; it is glad and lovely; it is strong, patient, and faithful; wise, longsuffering and resolute; it never seeks its own ends, for where a man seeks his own ends, he at once falls out of love. Love is sensible, humble, honorable; it is not self-indulgent, thoughtless, set on foolish things, but is sober, chaste, steadfast, quiet, and guarded in every sense. Love is submissive and obeys those set over it; for itself it has only disregard and contempt, but is full of devotion and gratitude to God; and it goes on trusting and hoping in God even when He is no longer sweet to it, for one cannot live in love without pain. Anyone who is not prepared to endure everything and to stand by the will of the Beloved is not worthy of the name of lover. A lover must gladly accept what is hard and bitter for the sake of the Beloved, and he must not have his allegiance shaken if hardships come his way.

From TAN Pubishing. "Thoughts of St. Therese." The chapter on Hope.

"Time is but a shadow, a dream; already God sees us in glory and takes joy in our eternal beatitude. How this thought helps my soul! I understand then why He lets us suffer."   VIII letter to her sister Celine.

"A Day . . . an hour . . . and we shall have reached the port! My God, what shall we see then? What is that life which shall never have an end? . . . Jesus will be the Soul of our soul. Unfathomable mystery*! 'Eye hath not seen, not ear heard, neither hath it entered into the heart of man what great things God hath prepared for them that love Him'. (I Cor. 2:9)* And this will all come soon—yes, very soon, if we ardently love Jesus." VI letter to her sister Celine.

"Life is passing, Eternity draweth nigh; soon shall we live the very life of God. After having drunk deep at the fount of bitterness, our thirst will be quenched at the very source of all sweetness.

Yes, *'the figure of this world passeth away" (1 Cor. 7:31),* soon shall we see new heavens' a more radiant sun will brighten with its splendors ethereal seas and infinite horizons . . . We shall no longer be prisoners in a land of exile, all will be at an end and with our Heavenly Spouse we shall sail over boundless waters; *now our harps are hung upon the willows that border the rivers of Babylon (Ps 136:2).* But in the day of our deliverance what harmonies will then be heard! With what joy shall we not make every chord of our instruments to vibrate! Today, *we weep remembering Sion . . . how shall we sing the songs of the Lord in a strange land? (Ps 136:4)."*   V letter to her sister Celine

"How I thirst for heaven—that blessed habitation where our love for Jesus will have no limit! But to get there we must suffer . . . we must weep . . . Well, I wish to suffer all that will please my beloved, I wish to do what He wills with his 'little ball' (she imagined herself as the Child Jesus' toy).   V letter to Sr. Marie of the Sacred Heart.

"OH! What mysteries will be revealed to us later . . . How often have I thought that I perhaps owe all the graces showered upon me to the earnest prayer of a little soul whom I shall know only in Heaven. It is God's will that in this world by means of prayer Heavenly treasures should be imparted by souls one to another, so that when they reach the Fatherland they may love one another with a love born of gratitude, with an affection far, far exceeding the most ideal family affection upon earth!

There, we shall meet with not indifferent looks! because all the Saints will be indebted to each other.

No envious glances will be seen; the happiness of everyone of the elect will be the happiness of all. With the Martyrs will shall be like to the Martyrs; with the Doctors we shall be as to the Doctors, with the Virgins as to the Virgins, and just as the members of a family are proud of one another, so shall we be of our brethren, without the least jealousy.

Who knows even if the joy we shall experience in beholding the glory of the greater Saints, and knowing that by a secret disposition of Providence we have contributed thereunto, who knows if this joy will not be as intense and sweeter perhaps, than the happiness they themselves will possess.

And do not think that on their side the great Saints, seeing what they owe to quite little souls, will love them with an incomparable love? Delightful and surprising will be the friendships found there—I am sure of it. The favored companion of an Apostle or a great Doctor of the church, will perhaps be a young shepherd lad; and a simple little child may be the intimate friend of a Patriarch. OH! How I long to dwell in that kingdom of Love . . . .
From: Counsels and Reminiscences.

From St. Ambrose . . . we are sons of God: we are heirs of God, co-heirs with Christ. A co-heir of Christ is one who is glorified along with Christ. The one who is glorified along with Him is one who by suffering for Him, suffers along with Him.

To encourage us in our suffering, Paul adds that all our sufferings are small in comparison with the wonderful reward that will be revealed in us; our labors do not deserve the blessings that are to come. We shall be restored to the likeness of God, and counted worthy of seeing Him face to face.

The following are scriptures I have used to help the dying, their families, and the family of recently deceased friends at funeral services I was asked to help with.

PSALMS: (From the NAB)

23 A Psalm of David. The Lord is my shepherd; there is nothing I lack. In green pastures You let me graze; to safe waters You lead me; You restore my strength. You guide me along the right path for the sake of Your name. Even when I walk through the dark valley, I fear no harm for You are at my side; Your rod and staff give me courage. You set a table before me as my enemies watch; You anoint my head with oil; my cup overflows. Only goodness and merciful love will pursue me all the days of my life; I will dwell in the house of the Lord for years to come.

Psalm 40, 42, 43 I waited, waited for the Lord; Who bent down and heard my cry, drew me out from the pit of destruction, out of the mud of the swamp, set my feet upon a rock, steadied my steps, and out a new song in my mouth, a hymn to our God. Many shall look on in awe and they shall trust in the Lord.

Happy those who trust in the Lord, who turn not to idolatry or to those who stray after falsehood. How numerous, O Lord, my God, You have made Your marvelous deeds! And in Your plans for us there is none to equal You. Shall I wish to tell or declare them, too many are they to recount.

Sacrifice and offering You do not want; but ears open to obedience You gave me. Holocausts and sin-offerings You do not require; so I said: "Here I am; Your commands for me are written in the scroll. To do Your will is my delight; my God Your law is in my heart!" I announced Your deed to a great assembly; I did not restrain my lips; You, Lord, are my witness. Your deed I did not hide within my heart; Your loyal deliverance I have proclaimed. I made no secret of Your enduring kindness to a great assembly.

Lord, do not withhold Your compassion from me; may Your enduring kindness ever preserve me. For all about me are evils beyond count; my sins so overcome me I cannot see. They are more than the hairs of my head; my courage fails me.

Lord, graciously rescue me! Come quickly to help me, Lord! Put to shame and confound all who seek to take my life. Turn back in disgrace those who desire my ruin. Let those who say, "Ah!" know dismay and shame. But may all who seek You rejoice and be glad in You. May those who long for Your help always say, "The Lord be glorified!" Though I am afflicted and poor, the Lord keeps me in my mind. You are help and deliverer; my God do not delay!

As the deer longs for streams of water, so my soul longs for You, O God. My being thirsts for God, the living God. When can I go and see the Face of God? My tears have been my food day and night, as they ask daily, "Where is Your God?" Those times I recall as I pour out my soul, when I went in procession with the crowd, I went with them to the house of God, Amid loud cries of thanksgiving, with the multitude keeping festival. Why are you downcast my soul; Why groan within me? Wait for God, whom I shall praise again, my savior and my God.

My soul is downcast within me; therefore I will remember You from the land of the Jordan and Hermon, from the land of Mount Mizar. Here deep calls to deep in the roar of Your torrents. All Your waves and breakers sweep over me. At dawn may the Lord bestow faithful love that I may sing praise through the night, praise to the God of my life. I say to God, "My Rock, why do You forget me? Why must I go about mourning with the enemy oppressing me?" It shatters my bones, when my adversaries reproach me. They say to me daily, "Where is your God?" Why are you downcast my soul; Why groan within me? Wait for God, whom I shall praise again, my savior and my God.

Grant me justice, God; defend me from a faithless people; from the deceitful and unjust rescue me. You, Go, are my strength. Why then do You spurn me? Why must I go about mourning with the enemy oppressing me? Send Your light and fidelity, that they might be my guide and bring me to Your holy mountain, to the place of Your dwelling, That I may come to the altar of God, to God, my joy, my delight. Then I will praise You with the harp, O god, my God. Why are you downcast my soul; Why groan within me? Wait for God, whom I shall praise again, my savior and my God.

Psalm 116 I love the LORD, who listened to my voice in supplication, Who turned an ear to me on the day I called. I was caught by the cords of death; the snares of Sheol had seized me; I felt agony and dread. Then I called on the name of the LORD, "O LORD, save my life!" Gracious is the LORD and just; yes, our God is merciful. The LORD protects the simple; I was helpless, but God saved me. Return, my soul, to your rest; the LORD has been good to you. For my soul has been freed from death, my eyes from tears, my feet from stumbling. I shall walk before the LORD in the land of the living.

I kept faith, even when I said, "I am greatly afflicted!" I said in my alarm, "No one can be trusted!" How can I repay the LORD for all the good done for me? I will raise the cup of salvation and call on the name of the LORD. I will pay my vows to the LORD in the presence of all his people. Too costly in the eyes of the LORD is the death of his faithful. LORD, I am your servant, your servant, the child of your maidservant; you have loosed my bonds. I will offer a sacrifice of thanksgiving and call on the name of the LORD. I will pay my vows to the LORD in the presence of all his people, In the courts of the house of the LORD, in your midst, O Jerusalem. Hallelujah!

Psalm 117 Praise the LORD, all you nations! Give glory, all you peoples! The LORD'S love for us is strong; the LORD is faithful forever. Hallelujah!

Psalm 112 A song of ascents. Of David. [1] I rejoiced when they said to me, "Let us go to the house of the LORD." And now our feet are standing within your gates, Jerusalem. Jerusalem, built as a city, walled round about. Here the tribes have come, the tribes of the LORD, As it was decreed for Israel, to give thanks to the name of the LORD. Here are the thrones of justice, the thrones of the house of David. For the peace of Jerusalem pray: "May those who love you prosper! May peace be within your ramparts, prosperity within your towers." For family and friends I say, "May peace be yours." For the house of the LORD, our God, I pray, "May blessings be yours."

Psalm 139: 1-24 For the leader. A psalm of David. O LORD, you have probed me, you know me: you know when I sit and stand; you understand my thoughts from afar. My travels and my rest you mark; with all my ways you are familiar. Even before a word is on my tongue, LORD, you know it all. Behind and before you encircle me and rest your hand upon me. Such knowledge is beyond me, far too lofty for me to reach. Where can I hide from your spirit? From your presence, where can I flee? If I ascend to the heavens, you are there; if I lie down in Sheol, you are there too. If I fly with the wings of dawn and alight beyond the sea, Even there your hand will guide me, your right hand hold me fast. If I say, "Surely darkness shall hide me, and night shall be my light"—

Darkness is not dark for you, and night shines as the day. Darkness and light are but one. You formed my inmost being; you knit me in my mother's womb. I praise you, so wonderfully you made me; wonderful are your works! My very self you knew; my bones were not hidden from you, When I was being made in secret, fashioned as in the depths of the earth. Your eyes foresaw my actions; in your book all are written down; my days were shaped, before one came to be. How precious to me are your designs, O God; how vast the sum of them! Were I to count, they would outnumber the sands; to finish, I would need eternity. If only you would destroy the wicked, O God, and the bloodthirsty would depart from me! Deceitfully they invoke your name; your foes swear faithless oaths. Do I not hate, LORD, those who hate you? Those who rise against you, do I not loathe? With fierce hatred I hate them, enemies I count as my own. Probe me, God, know my heart; try me, know my concerns. See if my way is crooked, then lead me in the ancient paths.

Ezekiel 37: 12-14 Therefore, prophesy and say to them: Thus says the Lord GOD: O my people, I will open your graves and have you rise from them, and bring you back to the land of Israel. Then you shall know that I am the LORD, when I open your graves and have you rise from them, O my people! I will put my spirit in you that you may live, and I will settle you upon your land; thus you shall know that I am the LORD. I have promised, and I will do it, says the LORD.

John 3: 14-16 And just as Moses lifted up the serpent in the desert, so must the Son of Man be lifted up, so that everyone who believes in him may have eternal life." For God so loved the world that he gave ^{z} his only Son, so that everyone who believes in him might not perish but might have eternal life.

John 6: 40 & 47 For this is the will of my Father, that everyone who sees the Son and believes in him may have eternal life, and I shall raise him (on) the last day." The Jews murmured about him because he said, "I am the bread that came down from heaven," and they said, "Is this not Jesus, the son of Joseph? Do we not know his father and mother? Then how can he say, 'I have come down from heaven'?" Jesus answered and said to them, "Stop murmuring among yourselves. No one can come to me unless the Father who sent me draw him, and I will raise him on the last day. It is written in the prophets: 'They shall all be taught by God.' Everyone who listens to my Father and learns from him comes to me. Not that anyone has seen the Father except the one who is from God; he has seen the Father. Amen, amen, I say to you, whoever believes has eternal life.

John 11: 25-30 Jesus told her, "I am the resurrection and the life; whoever believes in me, even if he dies, will live, and everyone who lives and believes in me will never die. Do you believe this?" She said to him, "Yes, Lord. I have come to believe that you are the Messiah, the Son of God, the one who is coming into the world." When she had said this, she went and called her sister Mary secretly, saying, "The teacher is here and is asking for you." As soon as she heard this, she rose quickly and went to him.

For Jesus had not yet come into the village, but was still where Martha had met him.

Roman 12: 1-2 I urge you therefore, brothers, by the mercies of God, to offer your bodies as a living sacrifice, holy and pleasing to God, your spiritual worship. Do not conform yourselves to this age but be transformed by the renewal of your mind, that you may discern what is the will of God, what is good and pleasing and perfect.

2 Corinthians 1: 3-7 Blessed be the God and Father of our Lord Jesus Christ, the Father of compassion and God of all encouragement, who encourages us in our every affliction, so that we may be able to encourage those who are in any affliction with the encouragement with which we ourselves are encouraged by God. For as Christ's sufferings overflow to us, so through Christ does our encouragement also overflow.

If we are afflicted, it is for your encouragement and salvation; if we are encouraged, it is for your encouragement, which enables you to endure the same sufferings that we suffer. Our hope for you is firm, for we know that as you share in the sufferings, you also share in the encouragement.

Philippians 3: 7-4: 1 & 4: 4-9 But) whatever gains I had, these I have come to consider a loss because of Christ. More than that, I even consider everything as a loss because of the supreme good of knowing Christ Jesus my Lord. For his sake I have accepted the loss of all things and I consider them so much rubbish, that I may gain Christ and be found in him, not having any righteousness of my own based on the law but that which comes through faith in Christ, the righteousness from God, depending on faith to know him and the power of his resurrection and (the) sharing of his sufferings by being conformed to his death, if somehow I may attain the resurrection from the dead.

It is not that I have already taken hold of it or have already attained perfect maturity, but I continue my pursuit in hope that I may possess it, since I have indeed been taken possession of by Christ (Jesus). Brothers, I for my part do not consider myself to have taken possession. Just one thing: forgetting what lies behind but straining forward to what lies ahead, I continue my pursuit toward the goal, the prize of God's upward calling, in Christ Jesus. Let us, then, who are "perfectly mature" adopt this attitude. And if you have a different attitude, this too God will reveal to you. Only, with regard to what we have attained, continue on the same course. Join with others in being imitators of me, brothers, and observe those who thus conduct themselves according to the model you have in us. For many, as I have often told you and now tell you even in tears, conduct themselves as enemies of the cross of Christ. Their end is destruction. Their God is their stomach; their glory is in their "shame." Their minds are occupied with earthly things. But our citizenship is in heaven, and from it we also await a savior, the Lord Jesus Christ. He will change our lowly body to conform with his glorified body by the power that enables him also to bring all things into subjection to himself. Therefore, my brothers, whom I love and long for, my joy and crown, in this way stand firm in the Lord, beloved.

4: 4-9 Rejoice in the Lord always. I shall say it again: rejoice! Your kindness should be known to all. The Lord is near. Have no anxiety at all, but in everything, by prayer and petition, with thanksgiving, make your requests known to God. Then the peace of God that surpasses all understanding will guard your hearts and minds in Christ Jesus.

Finally, brothers, whatever is true, whatever is honorable, whatever is just, whatever is pure, whatever is lovely, whatever is gracious, if there is any excellence and if there is anything worthy of praise, think about these things. Keep on doing what you have learned and received and heard and seen in me. Then the God of peace will be with you.

2 Thessalonians 1: 11-12 To this end, we always pray for you, that our God may make you worthy of his calling and powerfully bring to fulfillment every good purpose and every effort of faith, that the name of our Lord Jesus may be glorified in you, and you in him, in accord with the grace of our God and Lord Jesus Christ.

1 Peter 1: 17-21 Now if you invoke as Father him who judges impartially according to each one's works, conduct yourselves with reverence during the time of your sojourning, realizing that you were ransomed from your futile conduct, handed on by your

ancestors, not with perishable things like silver or gold but with the precious blood of Christ as of a spotless unblemished lamb. He was known before the foundation of the world but revealed in the final time for you, who through him believe in God who raised him from the dead and gave him glory, so that your faith and hope are in God.

From the Four Volume Liturgy of the Word
The Book of Wisdom
Chapter 1: 13-15

Because God did not make death, nor does he rejoice in the destruction of the living. For he fashioned all things that they might have being; and the creatures of the world are wholesome, And there is not a destructive drug among them nor any domain of the nether world on earth, For justice is undying. It was the wicked who with hands and words invited death, considered it a friend, and pined for it, and made a covenant with it, Because they deserve to be in its possession,

God has snatched me from the bonds of death, I shall walk among the living in His presence.

From the Tractates on the First Letter of John by St. Augustine (Tract. 4: PL35.) From the Four Volume Liturgy of the Hours.

The entire life of a good Christian is in fact an exercise of holy desire. You do not yet see what you long for, but the very act of desiring prepares you, so that when he comes you may see and be utterly satisfied.

Suppose you are going to fill some holder or container, and you know you will be given a large amount. Then you set about stretching your sack or wineskin or whatever it is. Why? Because you know the quantity you will have to put in it and your eyes tell you there is not enough room. By stretching it, therefore, you increase the capacity of the sack, and this is how God deals with us. Simply by making us wait he increases our desire, which in turn enlarges the capacity of our soul, making it able to receive what is to be given to us.

So, my brethren, let us continue to desire, for we shall be filled. Take note of Saint Paul stretching as it were his ability to receive what is to come: Not that I have already obtained this, he said, or am made perfect. Brethren, I do not consider that I have already obtained it. We might ask him, "If you have not yet obtained it, what are you doing in this life?" This one thing I do, answers Paul, forgetting what lies behind, and stretching forward to what lies ahead, I press on toward the prize to which I am called in the life above. Not only did Paul say he stretched forward, but he also declared that he pressed on toward a chosen goal. He realized in fact that he was still short of receiving what no eye has seen, nor ear heard, nor the heart of man conceived.

Such is our Christian life. By desiring heaven we exercise the powers of our soul. Now this exercise will be effective only to the extent that we free ourselves from desires leading to infatuation with this world. Let me return to the example I have already used, of filling an empty container. God means to fill each of you with what is good; so cast out what is bad! If he wishes to fill you with honey and you are full of sour wine, where is the honey to go? The vessel must be emptied of its contents and then be cleansed. Yes, it must be cleansed even if you have to work hard and scour it. It must be made fit for the new thing, whatever it may be.

We may go on speaking figuratively of honey, gold or wine—but whatever we say we cannot express the reality we are to receive. The name of that reality is God. But who will claim that in that one syllable we utter the full expanse of our heart's desire? Therefore, whatever we say is necessarily less than the full truth. We must extend ourselves toward the measure of Christ so that when he comes he may fill us with his presence. Then we shall be like him, for we shall see him as he is.

2 Corinthians 15: 12-57 (From the New American Bible, 1970, 2002—found in the Breviary or Liturgy of the Word)

But if Christ is preached as raised from the dead, how can some among you say there is no resurrection of the dead? If there is no resurrection of the dead, then neither has Christ been raised. And if Christ has not been raised, then empty (too) is our preaching; empty, too, your faith. Then we are also false witnesses to God, because we testified against God that he raised Christ, whom he did not raise if in fact the dead are not raised. For if the dead are not raised, neither has Christ been raised, and if Christ has not been raised, your faith is vain; you are still in your sins. Then those who have fallen asleep in Christ have perished.

If for this life only we have hoped in Christ, we are the most pitiable people of all. But now Christ has been raised from the dead, the first fruits of those who have fallen asleep. For since death came through a human being, the resurrection of the dead came also through a human being. For just as in Adam all die, so too in Christ shall all be brought to life, but each one in proper order: Christ the first fruits; then, at his coming, those who belong to Christ; then comes the end, when he hands over the kingdom to his God and Father, when he has destroyed every sovereignty and every authority and power. For he must reign until he has put all his enemies under his feet. The last enemy to be destroyed is death, for "he subjected everything under his feet." But when it says that everything has been subjected, it is clear that it excludes the one who subjected everything to him.

When everything is subjected to him, then the Son himself will (also) be subjected to the one who subjected everything to him, so that God may be all in all.

Otherwise, what will people accomplish by having themselves baptized for the dead? If the dead are not raised at all, then why are they having themselves baptized for them? Moreover, why are we endangering ourselves all the time? Every day I face death; I swear it by the pride in you (brothers) that I have in Christ Jesus our Lord. If at Ephesus I fought with beasts, so to speak, what benefit was it to me? If the dead are not raised: "Let us eat and drink, for tomorrow we die." Do not be led astray:

"Bad company corrupts good morals." Become sober as you ought and stop sinning. For some have no knowledge of God; I say this to your shame.

But someone may say, "How are the dead raised? With what kind of body will they come back?" You fool! What you sow is not brought to life unless it dies. And what you sow is not the body that is to be but a bare kernel of wheat, perhaps, or of some other kind; but God gives it a body as he chooses, and to each of the seeds its own body. Not all flesh is the same, but there is one kind for human beings, another kind of flesh for animals, another kind of flesh for birds, and another for fish. There are both heavenly bodies and earthly bodies, but the brightness of the heavenly is one kind and that of the earthly another. The brightness of the sun is one kind, the brightness of the moon another, and the brightness of the stars another. For star differs from star in brightness.

So also is the resurrection of the dead. It is sown corruptible; it is raised incorruptible. It is sown dishonorable; it is raised glorious. It is sown weak; it is raised powerful. It is sown a natural body; it is raised a spiritual body. If there is a natural body, there is also a spiritual one.

So, too, it is written, "The first man, Adam, became a living being," the last Adam a life-giving spirit. But the spiritual was not first; rather the natural and then the spiritual. The first man was from the earth, earthly; the second man, from heaven. As was the earthly one, so also are the earthly, and as is the heavenly one, so also are the heavenly. Just as we have borne the image of the earthly one, we shall also bear the image of the heavenly one. This I declare, brothers: flesh and blood cannot inherit the kingdom of God, nor does corruption inherit incorruption.

Behold, I tell you a mystery. We shall not all fall asleep, but we will all be changed, in an instant, in the blink of an eye, at the last trumpet. For the trumpet will sound, the dead will be raised incorruptible, and we shall be changed. For that which is corruptible must clothe itself with incorruptibility, and that which is mortal must clothe itself with immortality. And when this which is corruptible clothes itself with incorruptibility and this which is mortal clothes itself with immortality, then the word that is written shall come about: "Death is swallowed up in victory. Where, O death, is your victory? Where, O death, is your sting?" The sting of death is sin, and the power of sin is the law. But thanks be to God who gives us the victory through our Lord Jesus Christ.

Last Thoughts—From Brother Bernard Francis:

I know one who has seen a few of those who have died, and later reappeared to him in the beautiful, radiant, glorified, spiritual body. Some spoke, some merely smiled. What Paul and Jesus has foretold, he has seen with his own eyes. He said, "They are beautiful! More healthy and vibrant than one has ever seen or imagined them. They glow with a joy, a peace, a love, a knowledge of what He has prepared for us."

"It almost reminds me of seeing the Virgin Mary and her smile, O! her smile, all heaven in her smile!"

From a Letter of Saint Clare to Blessed Agnes of Prague—Breviary Vol. III.

. . . fix your gaze upon Him, meditate on Him, contemplate Him in your eagerness to imitate Him your loved one, the comeliest of men who became the vilest of men for your salvation, despised, buffeted, scourged and dying on the hard cross. If you suffer with Him, you shall reign with Him; if you mourn with Him, you shall rejoice with Him. If you die on the cross with Him in tribulations, you have an abode in heaven in the splendor of the Saints. Your name in the book of life will be glorious among men.

In recompense for this you will forever share in the glory of heaven in exchange for the fleeting things of earth, and in eternal possessions in exchange for those that perish. And you will live forever.

From Psalm 103 *For as the Heavens are high above the earth so strong is His love for those who fear Him. As far as the east is from the west so far does He remove our sins.*

From Judith 8: 25-27 *We should be grateful to our God, for putting us to the test, as He did our forefathers. Recall how He dealt with Abraham, and how He tried Isaac, and all that happened to Jacob in Syrian Mesopotamia while he was tending the flocks of Laban, his mother's brother. Not for vengeance did the Lord put them in the crucible to try their hearts, nor has He done so with us. It is by way of admonition that He chastises those who are close to Him.*

<u>From St. Gregory, Moral Reflections on Job</u>: *. . . We have this treasure in earthen vessels. Now in the blessed Job the earthen vessel felt gaping sores without, while this treasure of wisdom remained whole and intact within. Outwardly his body was in agony, but inwardly from the treasure of wisdom came holy thoughts: If we received good from the hand of the lord, why should we not endure evil? The good here refers to the temporal or eternal gifts of God, and the evil to the scourges of the present.*

. . . On the day of prosperity do not forget affliction, and on the day of affliction do not forget prosperity.

Saint John of the Cross would tell us, prosperity can lead to pride and abandoning God. But when we lose all, then He alone is our focus and our all.

<u>From St. Augustine's Confessions:</u> *Where did I find you, that I came to know You? You were not within my memory before I learned of You. Where, then, did I find You before I came to know You, if not within Yourself, far above me? We come to You and go from You, but no place is involved in this process. In every place, O Truth, You are present to those who seek Your help, and at one and the same time You answer all, though they seek Your counsel on different matters.*

You respond clearly, but not everyone hears clearly. All ask what they wish, but do not always hear the answer they wish. Your best servant is he who is intent not so much on hearing his petition answered, as rather on willing what he hears from You.

Late have I loved You, O Beauty ever ancient, ever new, late have I loved You! You were within me, but I was outside, and it was there that I searched for You . . .

When once I shall be united to You with my whole being, I shall at last be free from sorrow and toil. Then my life will be alive, filled entirely with You.

St. Teresa of the Andes: from <u>God the Joy of My Life</u> by Michael D. Griffin, OCD

She said that Our Lord told her: "if you want to be like Me, then take up your cross with love and joy." Moved by these words, she explains the deep reasons that drew her to seek suffering: *"Suffering pleases me so much for two reasons: because Jesus preferred suffering from His birth until His death on the cross. It must then be something very great since the All-Powerful One sought to suffer always. And suffering also pleases me because it is in the crucible of sorrow that souls are formed and because Jesus gives this gift to those He loves the most."* She wanted to become, *"a victim soul. To suffer to save souls & aid in the sanctification of priests."*

Brother Bernard Francis, SFO: I was feeling a bit down about my problems sometimes focusing my thoughts and remembering where I put things. This is a new problem for me these past 12 months. My wife said, "You are concerned about your mind? Your thinking? You've written several journal articles and five books!" I repented of my getting down for a moment for this too is a suffering that can be accepted with joy as a treasure that can be offered up for poor souls. So I thanked God for it, told Him I would gladly suffer it, and offered it up for the poor souls and sinners, and priests.

Then I reflected on what she had said. It was not true. Oh, I had written the words down, and they had gotten published and had helped others. But, you see, when ever we have a talent, or do good to others, these are God! It is His using us to help us and His children. I am nothing. I was a C-D student nearly my whole life until at 21 I found Him, then miraculously I became an A with a few B's student.

Every journal article, every book I have written I prayed to God <u>first</u>. I asked Him should I write this, will it accomplish good? I asked Him to help me to write it for, "You know I am not smart and not good with words." Funny I read of Moses saying the same thing re: pharaoh just yesterday morning: "How can I talk to him. You know I am poor with words."

I so well remember my first book. God told me to write it. I replied I can't write a book. He can be very persuasive. I asked Him to help and guide me and He did. When I read it I honestly thought "Wow! This is really good." It was as if I had nothing to do with it. As if God Himself had written it and I was reading it for the first time. Truly!

It has been this way with every book since. He has said, "Write this!" I have asked Him to guide my mind and hand. Mary to protect me from distractions, Therese to edit and help me rhyme. I am always amazed at how when I pray for His help each day I return to the writing, how He will order me to go and start and then reveal throughout my days what He wants added, what to write next. They are truly not my books at all. They are His books. I am simply the pencil. Remember the quote in the beginning of the book,

"I am nothing. A pencil can do nothing by itself. It needs a hand, strength and a mind to use it. God so often chooses the least worthy (St. Francis' words), the most ignorant (St. Bernadette's words). Then His power and His will use this instrument to accomplish His purpose out of love for His children. Then His love is seen and embraced. It is all God. How blessed to be an instrument in His hand. How blessed to know and love Him and to be content whether in His hand, or lying on the table awaiting His will." Bro. Bernard Francis, SFO

You need as the reader to know who the true author is. God, your loving Father. If these books have blessed you, then that is from Him. Any typographical errors etc. you find, those are mine, I don't always listen as well as I want to. My experiences with the dying and disabled? His, He guided me to be a nurse, helped me work with them, talk with them and help them, brought me into contact with various practitioners, years before I ever thought of writing a book.

All my books are available through AuthorHouse.com. Their address: Author House 1663 Liberty Drive, Bloomington IN 47403. Phone: 1-888-519-5121. In the past they have also been available through Barnes & Noble and Amazon bookstores.

1) Leadership in The Heat of Battle-2004, 2) Saints Francis of Assisi and Therese of Lisieux. My Companions on the Journey—2010, 3) Saints Francis of Assisi, and

Therese of Lisieux and Bernadette. My Companions on the Journey—2010, 4) Saints Francis of Assisi and Therese of Lisieux and Other Saints. My Companions on the Journey, Through the Dark Night into the Eternal Day—2010, 5) The White Chapel . . .—2011.

The first one I wrote on my own time, the last four were written while I worked as a consultant for the <u>Ian Clark Foundation DBA Therese's Missions</u>, a non-profit Catholic Charitable organization. Phone: 937-313-7290. These four belong to them as I worked on these to aid in their mission of making others aware of God's love and to make Him much loved.

It is our hope you will be blessed by each of these.

This book resulted from the requests of family care givers for a talk about death and dying. They were losing a loved and wanted to know what to expect.

As nurse practitioner I gained insights from Oncology Nurses, Hospice Nurses and Critical Care Nurses on how to help terminal patients obtain the most out of their remaining time. I went from a fear of talking with those dying, to feeling blessed to share this intimate time with them.

After 41 years of nursing, research and lecturing on this subject I began to understand, as I applied my own suffering from a disabling illness, of the comfort available from the Communion of Saints. Especially from those who said yes to God's request they suffer and join this suffering to that of His Son to help other souls, out of love for Him. Through my experiences with loved ones, patients and myself, I found tremendous help in turning to the Bible and the writings of Saints.

This book is a blending of spiritual hope & frank facts regarding suffering & dying that it is my prayer will bring strength to patents & care givers, be they physicians, nurses, aides or family.

www.ingramcontent.com/pod-product-compliance
Lightning Source LLC
Chambersburg PA
CBHW020249290526
45784CB00003B/1167